The Back
to
Basics Diet

The Back
to
Basics Diet

or

Seven Weeks to Change Your Life

The remarkable, groundbreaking guide to safe,
effective weight loss based on modern science
and the fascinating story of human evolution

David R Hack

Matador
9 Priory Business Park,
Wistow Road, Kibworth Beauchamp,
Leicestershire. LE8 0RX
Tel: 0116 279 2299
Email: books@troubador.co.uk
Web: www.troubador.co.uk/matador
Twitter: @matadorbooks

ISBN 9781788034395

British Library Cataloguing in Publication Data.
A catalogue record for this book is available from the British Library.

Printed in the UK by CPI Ltd, Croyden, UK
Typeset in Adobe Garamond by Troubador Publishing Ltd

Matador® is an imprint of Troubador Publishing Ltd

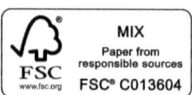

To Carol, the love of my life.
DH

DISCLAIMER

The ideas and concepts in this book are for information and educational-purposes only and do not constitute medical advice. This book is sold on the understanding that the author is not offering medical advice nor attempting to replace the advice of a doctor or other health care professional. It is vital that before beginning any diet or exercise programme, including the Back to Basics Diet, you receive clearance and guidance from your doctor or other appropriate health professional.

The decision to follow any information in this book remains solely the discretion of the reader, who does so of their own free will and assumes full responsibility for any or all consequences arising from such a decision. The author is not responsible for any specific health or allergy needs that may require medical supervision and is not liable for any loss, damages or negative consequences that might arise directly or indirectly from the use, application or interpretation of the material in this book. References are provided for informational purposes only and do not constitute endorsement of any websites or other sources.

Contents

Foreword

Eddy Marshall

On the morning of the 28th of January 2015, I popped in to my local doctor's surgery to learn the results of a blood test. I wasn't even vaguely prepared for what I was about to be told.

Although I'd been overweight for years, I remained reasonably fit and well, or so I thought. I definitely wasn't expecting my stony-faced GP to inform me that I had *advanced* Type 2 diabetes, requiring immediate medication and some stern doctorly admonishment.

At that point, I didn't know much about Type 2 diabetes (T2D) but the little I did know didn't fill me with joy.

I knew T2D meant as many as 10 years struck from my life expectancy, a sobering thought, especially for a happily married man with a four year-old son. That said, death might be considered a blessing if presaged by some of T2D's many awful comorbidities, including blindness, nerve-death, amputation and a far greater likelihood of heart attack, cancer and stroke. I knew T2D could well mean a creeping, unpleasant and premature decline.

Fortunately, things turned out to be a little less dark than I'd first thought and over the following week I learned a lot of new information about the condition.

In the week following my diagnosis, my wife Claire

ordered a copy of Dr David Cavan's *Reverse Your Diabetes*, which provided invaluable information and also hope that my T2D perhaps wasn't as intractable as I – and my GP – first thought. A couple of days after that, we purchased a copy of the 2014 edition of *The Back To Basics Diet*.

I went on to lose 50 pounds over the next five months, by changing my diet to something pretty close to the one advocated in this book. Just over a year after my diagnosis I was signed off my surgery's Diabetic Register, unmedicated and with no remaining indication of the condition.

The reversal of my T2D rests largely on these two books.

There's little similarity between the food I eat now compared to what I ate pre-T2D diagnosis. I now eat more consciously and with more relish and enjoyment than I ever did before diagnosis.

Inevitably (and logically), the free market has provided us with an ample choice of foods which are appealing and thus profitable but, because of their often essentially sugary/carby components, are also frequently unhealthy, even addictive. The consequent extremely poor health outcomes, with mass overweight and burgeoning T2D, have led to some equally extreme dietary 'cures' and in the midst of all this we've lost track of a lot of older wisdom regarding food, fasting, diet and health.

The Back to Basics Diet redresses that, bringing the essential truth about food back to the fore: that the food we eat ought to, first and foremost, nourish us.

In the course of making an ongoing film on the subject of T2D reversal, I was delighted to discover that David Hack is a fellow Cumbrian and near neighbour of mine, living a mere 20 miles away. Since then, David has helped out with some of our group work on T2D reversal, giving our participants lucid and witty talks on diet and evolution.

I recommend *The Back to Basics Diet* very highly indeed. Too many of us have been taught too little about these most basic facts of life, about the right foods to eat for our best health and wellbeing.

This book is necessary and timely and I hope you gain as much insight, good health and enjoyment from it as I have.

Eddy Marshall
Grange-over-Sands, September 2017
TV Director & Co-Founder of *Dia-Beat This!*
Type 2 diabetes reversal course and film.

Welcome to The Back to Basics Diet 2018 edition

I first published *The Back to Basics Diet* in 2014 and since then have been delighted with the overwhelmingly positive response to the book. Unfortunately, the world of nutrition and obesity research never sleeps, so in an effort to keep things up to date I thought it would be sensible to update the book for 2018.

I decided to sit down and write a diet book some years ago when I was going through a difficult and challenging phase of my life. Notwithstanding my own personal troubles, one day, when I was at a particularly low ebb, I stood alone in front of my bedroom mirror and got the shock of my life. Somehow, I had become really fat. To make matters worse, my doctor told me I was suffering from numerous obesity-related problems, i.e. disruptive sleep apnea, hypertension (high blood pressure) and pre-diabetes. I was stunned; if I carried on in this way, I was headed for a lifetime of illness and an early grave. How on Earth had I got myself into this state?

I grew up eating home-cooked food prepared by my mum, who like many women of her era had grown up during the War and so was adept at making ends meet. My parents had lived abroad before they married, so mealtimes included wonderful curries (my father had lived in India during the War) and Mediterranean foods inspired by the years my mother had spent in Europe. Together with lots of sport at school, this home-cooked, real food diet kept me healthy and slim.

Unfortunately, after leaving home, the dietary wheels began to fall off. Mealtimes became dominated by takeaways and beer, so slowly but surely I began to put on weight. However, it was to be many years later before I finally took that long, hard look in the mirror. At this point I had reached nearly seventeen stone (240 pounds), almost 50% over my ideal weight. Enough was enough.

Desperate for answers to my declining health and gripped by a severe mid-life crisis, I took myself off to university in search of the answers to my rapidly declining health. Over the next few years, I learned about human biology, biochemistry, anatomy and human evolution before the answer I had been searching for started to emerge. In fact, it wasn't long before I realized that the solution to my ever-increasing waistline was staring me in the face; I finally knew how you and I are *designed* to eat.

We have all been led a merry dance towards a lifetime of obesity and ill health by the very foods we put in our mouths each and every day. It is time to change that now, once and for all. In fact, we need to look at our diet and lifestyle from a completely new perspective, which is what this book is all about.

I sincerely hope the Back to Basics diet will change your life, for better and forever.

Introduction

Better a diamond with a flaw than a pebble without.
Confucius

Welcome to the Back to Basics diet, the proven weight loss system based on modern science and the fascinating story of human evolution. There are no gimmicks here, just a straightforward explanation as to why a plant-based, real food diet and gentle daily exercise holds the key to successful weight loss.

To understand why so many of us struggle with our weight, we need to take a peak into our evolutionary past and have a brief look at the nuts and bolts of how we digest our food. In so doing, we soon uncover the real reasons behind our expanding waistlines and how we can fix that, once and for all. Along the way, we will discover the secret of *what* and *when* to eat to ensure we both lose weight and keep that weight off for life. And as we will see, this is a far cry from how many of us eat today.

By making the changes recommended in this book, remarkable things happen. Weight loss becomes effortless, our health receives a huge boost and we give ourselves the best possible chance of fending off modern lifestyle diseases such as Type 2 diabetes. This is in complete contrast to the majority of diets where we are expected to live on tiny portions of food in order to lose weight; eventually, we get so hungry we just can't cope any more and in desperation reach for the nearest cream cake. That won't happen here because the Back to Basics diet contains real, natural foods that are filling and satisfying, so hunger pangs disappear and we soon lose the desire to eat the comfort foods that got us in this state in the first place. Losing weight just becomes a happy by-product of a satisfying and healthy diet, with no overpowering urge to return to eating cakes. Better still, we save money eating this way, too.

Why Back to Basics?

The Back to Basics diet involves a fundamental change to the way we eat, away from a toxic, sugar-laden, processed food diet to our natural diet, the diet we are designed to eat as healthy human beings. As we will see, this natural diet is very much a *plant-based* diet, not a meat-heavy 'Paleo' or 'Caveman' diet. Such diets may be on the right track (e.g. no processed carbohydrate) but we can't escape the fact that we are designed, by evolution, to eat a predominantly plant-based diet.

By returning to our natural diet, we will again be eating in accordance with our evolutionary design. This in itself allows us to re-build our skewed relationship with food and sets the wheels in motion for successful weight loss.

Are we really too big these days?

There is little doubt that we are living in the midst of an obesity epidemic.[1] Across the globe, obesity levels have never been higher and we humans are fatter now than at any time in our history.[2] Regardless of the reasons behind all this, if you or I visit the doctor, he or she can work out whether or not we are underweight, of normal weight or overweight/obese by using something called the Body Mass Index (BMI). This is a mathematical relationship that relates our weight to our height. In the UK, the BMI score is calculated as follows:

BMI (kg/m2)	Description
Less than 18.5	Underweight
18.5 to less than 25	Normal
25 to less than 30	Overweight
30 or more	Obese
40 or more	Morbidly obese

Fifty years ago, a doctor would have had very little obesity-related work. Things are very different today in the UK, where large numbers of adults and children are now classed as technically overweight or obese.[3] In fact, obesity levels are rapidly getting out of control; in 2015, the NHS calculated that 27% of all adults in England were obese, whilst 41% of men and 31% of women were overweight.[4]

Obesity is a worldwide problem

We are certainly getting bigger in the UK but things are much worse in the USA, which can lay dubious claim to being the home of obesity. A couple of years ago, roughly 35% of all Americans were classed as clinically obese.[5] However, if things continue as they are, all adults in the US will be obese by 2048.[6]

Does any of this matter? Isn't our body shape our business? Well, maybe, but obesity is a leading cause of Type 2 diabetes and heart disease and is associated with a number of cancers, too.[7] The link between Type 2 diabetes and obesity is so well established that many doctors use the phrase 'diabesity' to refer to these two inter-linked conditions.[8] Obesity can also lead to depression and an increase in dementia and is also hugely expensive to treat; in the UK alone, the cost of obesity treatment could reach almost £50 billion per annum by 2050.[9]

Rich or poor – obesity doesn't care

For much of human history, only the wealthy could afford to eat enough to get fat. However, nowadays it seems that obesity is somehow linked to poverty.[10] There are numerous complex reasons for this which are outside the scope of this book, but sadly it is often the poorest sections of society who present with the highest rates of obesity.[11,12] This is a very complex issue but there seems little doubt that the availability of high-calorie, low-nutrient fast foods play a major part in the obesity epidemic, particularly amongst the young and the poorer members of our society.[13,14,15]

Our problematic relationship with food

Food is something that should be cherished and enjoyed

but these days it seems that our relationship with food has fundamentally broken down. In the developed world, we suffer from so many obesity-related diseases our healthcare systems are struggling to cope; meanwhile, the images of malnourished and starving children in the world's poorest regions break our hearts.[2] Despite these two extremes, our own relationship with food suffers due to our hectic lives and the availability of foods 24/7, most of which are a long way from being the natural foods we are designed to eat. In terms of *our* overweight and obesity, we can lay the blame firmly at the door of our over-caloried, modern diet.

The good news is that healthy eating is within the grasp of each and every one of us, regardless of our wealth or health status. Nevertheless, if we abdicate responsibility for what we eat to the nearest takeaway (or garage forecourt shop or that nice lady with the trolley on the train), we are in danger of an inexorable drift towards the famous slippery slope and a lifetime of obesity and ill health. Instead, by adopting a true Back to Basics diet – i.e. a real food, predominantly plant-based diet, we can begin to lose weight, improve our health and start to feel much better about the world around us and about ourselves as well.

It is time to look after Number One

The science that follows in this book underpins our new, healthy diet (and can tell us why so many of us are overweight and how we can fix it) but science alone can't resolve our weight problems. For that to happen, we need to start putting ourselves first in life; in fact, to lose weight successfully, we need to look after Number One.

None of us is naturally selfish, so it is only human nature to put everything that is important to us (e.g. careers, partners, children, social life) before our own needs each and every day. However, to make real, lasting changes to our weight and health, we have to consider our needs first. This means we have to think about *our* meals and *our* daily routine first, before getting on with everything else in life. Putting ourselves front and centre like this is the first step in regaining control of our relationship with food and sets us up for successful weight loss.

Changing lives for the better

Many of the foods available to us today are so far removed from those we evolved to eat that it is hardly surprising so many of us struggle with our weight. Despite our best efforts, the odds of staying healthy and slim are stacked against us and without some specialist knowledge it is very easy to lose control of sensible eating habits, as many of us know to our cost. Unfortunately, much of what we find on our supermarket shelves is designed to maximize profit for the food industry, not necessarily to make us healthy or slim. That's why ditching the damaging junk food of our modern food environment is so important; we can then make the change to a plant-based, real food diet and move on with our lives in a far healthier way.

Most diets fail because the dieter eventually gets *so*

hungry, he or she can no longer ignore the natural human instinct to eat. However, on a real food, plant-based diet we get to eat plenty of food, so we never feel deprived or hungry. If we can also make some subtle changes to *when* we eat and embrace the idea of getting active every day, we can lose weight steadily and effortlessly and without the fear of starvation, so common on traditional diets. Even if we have the odd wobble or fall off the diet wagon for a while, we just need to pick ourselves up and carry on where we left off. No pressure or recriminations, just another gentle reboot of our diet and lifestyle so that we can again start to lose weight.

The Back to Basics Diet is a template for life

If you have tried every diet in the book with little success, don't beat yourself up because you are most definitely not alone; it is almost impossible to lose weight effectively on traditional diets. Instead, we need a way to lose weight that works in harmony with how we are designed to function as healthy human beings. The Back to Basics diet provides just this sort of approach to weight loss. Full of healthy eating tips and tricks and a foolproof step-by-step system, the programme helps re-establish a healthy relationship with real food and re-calibrates our lives so that we can again be in tune with how we are meant to eat. All we need is a gentle push in the right direction and the right tools for the job – which is what this book is all about.

A famous nutritionist once said, "Human nutrition isn't rocket science, you know? No, it is much, much more complicated than that!" He was right, too. Nevertheless, by following a simple, straightforward plan such as the Back to Basics diet, we can give ourselves the best possible chance of losing weight once and for all.

PART ONE

1

Is it our fault we get fat?

It is time to challenge the status quo

A well-meaning doctor or other health professional might tell us that our excess weight is due to over-eating, coupled to a lack of exercise. In other words, we are eating too many calories compared to the number of calories we need (because we don't exercise much), so we put on weight.[1] If they are kind, they will break this news gently; if not, they will leave us in little doubt that our excess weight is simply down to greed and laziness. This is the reality we all face today in a world where obesity is regarded as a self-inflicted disease, i.e. our obesity is our fault.[2,3] The consensus is that obesity is simply a matter of 'calories in – calories out', a view not helped by the fact that those of us who are overweight often appear to eat more than thin people. And yes, overweight and obese people find it hard to take exercise in a practical sense, even if they have the inclination to do so.

We need a more understanding approach to obesity

The idea that obesity is somehow 'our fault' is not only unjust but also plain wrong in scientific terms, too.[4] In fact,

NEED TO KNOW

- Our modern diet makes it almost impossible to lose weight through willpower alone.
- The foods we eat today contain unnaturally high levels of calories and disturb various chemical signals (hormones) inside our bodies, resulting in almost continuous weight gain and an uncontrollable urge to eat.
- Re-establishing a healthy relationship with real food allows our hormone systems to return to sensitivity – we will no longer be swimming against the tide of our own body chemistry.
- Eating real food and changing when we eat will allow effortless weight loss. No willpower required!

overweight is caused primarily by the *types* of foods we eat as part of our modern diet.[5] These unnatural foods cause changes in chemical systems inside our body, such that we constantly try to store the energy from food in the form of fat. At the same time, we don't recognize the signals that are desperately telling us we have eaten enough so stop eating. Consequently, we do eat too many calories and then store much of the food we eat as fat. That's why it is quite wrong to suggest that we should all pull ourselves together or otherwise use old-fashioned willpower to lose weight when our body chemistry is so damaged by our modern diet.[6,7]

If our obesity is not our fault, what then is the solution to our weight issues? We will look at this in some detail in the following chapters but in essence, the key to *permanent* weight loss (as opposed to the dreaded yo-yo dieting) is to change *what* and *when* we eat, so that we can start to re-establish a healthy relationship with food. In doing so, we will consume fewer calories and so lose weight safely and effortlessly and improve our health at the same time. We will become sensitive to chemical signals that tell us when we are 'full' (and so won't eat too many calories at each meal) and will use our food to fuel the cells, tissues and organs of our body, rather than storing it as fat all the time. This is the essence of the Back to Basics diet – by eating real food at the appropriate times of the day, we can naturally reduce our calorie intake and regain sensitivity to our body's various chemical signals. By returning to a natural, real food diet, we have no need to dramatically restrict portion size, either. Obesity is not our fault – it's all down to the types of food we used to eat in the bad old days.

Our hormones hold the key

Most of the chemical signals sent haywire by our modern diet are hormones of one sort or another. When we change the way our bodies react to these hormones through the types of food we eat, it is difficult to avoid putting on weight, even if we count calories or try to use huge amounts of will power to eat less food. Similarly, we will never lose weight successfully by eating small portions of modern, processed foods (the basis for most diets) because it is impossible to stick to such restrictive diets for very long before we fall off the wagon.

Stressed out? Suffer from food addictions?

THE BACK TO BASICS DIET CAN HELP

- Stressed, lonely or anxious? Do you crave sweet or fatty foods?
- When we are stressed, our body produces a hormone called cortisol, which is directly related to obesity. High levels of cortisol increase cravings for sugar and fat.
- To try to manage stress, it helps to get active in the fresh air or take up yoga, Tai Chi or other form of meditation.
- We could all do with putting ourselves first in life as well, now and again. We need to be mindful of our own health and happiness.
- The Back to Basics diet helps control cortisol levels by encouraging a switch to a real food diet, the odd glass of red wine rather than regular boozing and daily activity outside in the fresh air.

Our modern diet, comprising highly processed foods, upsets these hormonal systems such that we become resistant to the signals the hormones are trying to send.[8] For instance, if we are resistant to the hormonal signal that tells us we are full and have eaten enough, we instead suffer from an uncontrollable urge to eat.

So, over-eating, meaning we eat too many calories and hence gain weight, is mostly down to the type of food we eat. Many of us have grown up eating highly processed foods, which give us more calories than we really need and upset various hormone systems that lead directly to weight gain.

We will look at our 'food hormones' (primarily insulin and leptin) in more detail later but if these particular hormones are disturbed or become ineffective because of the types of food we eat, it is very hard, if not impossible, to lose any weight at all.[9,10]

We are meant to eat real food

In the Back to Basics diet, food is categorized as either 'real' or 'processed' food. We will have a look at real foods in much greater detail later because they underpin all the dietary changes I recommend in Part 2. However, real food is mainly the food that sustained our ancestors over hundreds of thousands of years before the invention of agriculture, e.g. small amounts of natural (ideally organic) meat, poultry, eggs and fish plus plenty of fruit, vegetables, salads, some tubers and nuts etc.[11] There are a few modern foods that also fit perfectly with Back to Basics eating and I'll cover those as we go along as well.

Real foods provide us with all the nutrients we require but contain relatively few calories. A diet of real foods forms the basis of the ideal human diet, one that allows us to lose weight and improve our health forever more.

Processed food – the real villain of the story

Unfortunately, much of the food we are offered in the supermarket or when eating out consists of heavily processed foods, not real food. Rather than going from the farmer's field (or from the butcher or fishmonger) directly to our dinner plate, what starts out as real food ends up being processed in a factory before being sold to us as myriad forms of convenience foods. Such foods provide economic benefit to the food industry but often bear little resemblance to the real, natural foods we are designed to eat. A list of such foods would fill a separate book but they are mainly the products of agriculture that are turned into mass-produced food right around the globe, e.g. fast food takeaways, supermarket ready meals, sweets, crisps, snacks, fizzy drinks, white bread, white rice, pasta, processed meats and fish, various low-fat products.

These processed foods tend to give us very little, if any, nutritional benefit but contain bucket loads of calories.[12] Coupled to a lack of exercise, a processed food diet invariably means we consume too many calories and so we will put on weight. Similarly, eating the worst examples of these foods means we are denying ourselves the wonderful array of nutrients contained in real food, which are essential for staving off numerous nasty diseases and ensuring we have a long and healthy life.

Changing mindsets

We all have dark days when we don't really care that much

about our weight or the damage it is doing to our health. It is easy to ignore the warnings from our friends and family (let alone from our doctor) and put our head in the sand, rather than doing something about it. Sometimes, we might not care that much about ourselves at all. I speak from experience as I spent much of my adult life ignoring my ever-expanding waistline and the damage my rather chaotic diet and lifestyle was doing to my health. I am nothing if not honest, so I would be lying if I said life was all plain sailing after that episode with the mirror. Nevertheless, the process of working out the nuts and bolts of the Back to Basics diet has been cathartic and has opened my own eyes to the simple dietary changes that make such a huge difference, not only to our waistlines but to our health and sense of self-esteem as well.

By switching to a real food diet and getting active, we can lose weight and change our health for the better, once and for all. There are other tips and tricks to learn along the way but it is remarkable how life can improve by just making these two simple (if fundamental) changes. The food industry is only doing its job but it is foolish to think their primary motive is to care about our health. They will huff and puff about why their products are good for us but at the end of the day, they are in the business of making a profit, not being our health advisor. It is up to us to decide what we eat and how much activity we should take – no one else. All we need to make the correct choices is some nutritional guidance, a basic understanding of what is really happening to us when we eat certain foods and a structured plan to ease us into a new, healthy way of eating. Well, that's all here in the pages of this book. In the meantime, let's see why, ultimately, diets just don't work.

2

Why diets just don't work

It is the mark of an educated mind to entertain
a thought without accepting it.
Aristotle

Eating less and moving more

Doctors and other health professionals keep telling us to 'eat less and move more' in an attempt to help us lose weight and improve our health.[1] Such advice is undoubtedly well meaning but it has singularly failed to reduce the current epidemic of obesity which, as we know, increases year on year.

To lose weight we need to eat fewer calories but simply eating less modern, processed food is not the answer.[2] We get precious little nutrition with this type of food in the first place; simply eating less of it just reduces our nutrient intake even further. Reducing our portion size will mean we eat fewer calories but, as we all know, it is impossible to stick to such restrictive diets for more than a few weeks, at best.

What about 'moving more'? This is excellent advice and burning more calories through exercise will certainly help us to lose weight, provided we eat properly as well.[3]

Unfortunately, many of us view exercise as something we either avoid at all costs or perhaps dabble in once or twice a week, when we take the dog out for a walk or play with the kids in the garden. Simply 'moving more' will have little, if any, effect on reducing our waistlines unless we can make some fundamental changes to our diet as well.[4]

The diet industry is full of contradictions

It is hardly surprising we are so confused about which diet to follow when we are faced with a constant barrage of dietary advice, such as eat 'low fat, high carb' or 'high carb, low fat' or 'no fat at all', 'low-carb', 'no carb' etc – what on Earth are we supposed to eat? Are carbs good or bad? Should we eat more or less protein? What about fat? If it's any comfort, the scientists and medical professionals are often confused as well.[5] To find the answer to this conundrum, we need to strip everything back to basics to see why most diets simply don't work.

We canna change the laws of physics, Captain

We humans are just a very small part of all the living and non-living elements that make up our known Universe. Whether we like it or not, we are all governed by the Laws of Physics, those sums we did our best to avoid at school. Some of these Laws relate to whether or not we put on weight, including the Law which states that 'energy can neither be created nor destroyed' and the Law which states that the amount of energy we are able to store in our bodies as fat is equal to the amount of energy in the food we eat minus the energy used doing work or otherwise lost to the Universe as something called entropy, e.g. heat. No more physics, I promise.

In terms of our weight, this means that:

CHANGE IN BODY FAT =
ENERGY CONSUMED – ENERGY BURNED
(calories in)   (calories out)

The experts argue endlessly over whether or not these particular Laws apply to us at all, particularly in terms of our ability to lose or put on weight.[6] I think they do. Some researchers believe that "a calorie is not a calorie", which in some ways is true.[7] This mostly relates to the effects of dietary sugar, which we will consider in more detail when we look at sugar as a foodstuff later.

Do calories really matter?

A calorie is simply a unit of measurement (of heat energy) and a way for food scientists to list the energy content of various foods. Nowadays, many diets encourage us to forget all about calories, often with mixed results. I don't fixate on calories in the Back to Basics diet because the recommended dietary changes (to a real food diet) create an inherently low calorie diet, so the calories look after themselves. Nevertheless, there is no escaping the fact that if we eat more calories than we burn up in any given time period, we will put on weight.[8]

There is no harm in counting calories, so if you want to be methodical in your approach have a look at the Basal Metabolic Rate (BMR) sums in Appendix 1. However, my recommended meal plans, daily activity suggestion and tips and tricks in Part 2 will help get calorie intake under control effortlessly, meaning we don't actually have to count calories ever again.

Calorie consumption is the over-arching factor in all discussions about weight loss. Nevertheless, the secret to losing weight and giving our health a huge boost involves changes to our diet and lifestyle that are easy to do but go much further than simply 'eating less and moving more'.

Dieting is not the answer

If losing weight was simply a question of eating fewer calories, why aren't we all slim?[9] Millions of people take up a new diet each year, only to fall off the wagon a few weeks later, even if they have lost some weight in the meantime. The reason most diets fail is because we get hungry. If we try to lose weight on a diet of modern, processed foods, we need to eat tiny portions in order to restrict our calorie intake. We will certainly eat fewer calories but such tiny portions make it impossible to stick to the diet in question for very long before the constant hunger becomes unbearable. Eventually, we can't stand it any more and reach for the nearest cake. Sound familiar?

Some diets also risk us eventually succumbing to malnutrition. A diet entirely comprising the worst examples of processed foods (but in tiny portions) runs the risk of reducing the amount of nutrients we eat to dangerously low levels.[10] Any form of restriction diet, by its very nature, is liable to lead to inadequate nutrition, even if it is effective in achieving short-term weight loss. Add the fact that most of us who eat a typical 'Western diet' are not getting enough life-enhancing nutrients in the first place and we are in a whole heap of trouble.[11] The Back to Basics diet approaches the idea of calorie restriction and healthy eating in a completely new way.[12,13] By replacing modern, processed foods with plentiful, healthy, real food and eating at the right time of day (when our body is naturally primed to use that food, rather than ready to store it as fat), we will naturally eat fewer calories and our portion sizes will be quite normal, so we won't get hungry. We can then lose weight effortlessly without resorting to willpower and give our health a huge boost at the same time.

Weight loss and health – a complete package

Let's imagine we have been invited to observe the goings on in a specialist food lab, where a volunteer has just arrived for a dietary experiment. Our volunteer is a 40-year-old female, five feet five inches tall and weighing 200 pounds (14.3 stones). If we were to get technical and use the BMR sums, we would discover that she has to eat approximately 2000 calories each day to sustain her normal life; to lose weight, she needs to eat slightly fewer calories or burn up more calories through exercise.

Back in the lab, our volunteer is offered the choice of one of two sets of meals (breakfast, lunch, dinner) for the day, both of which contain the same number of calories. In other words, it doesn't matter whether she chooses to eat her meals from the first group (Group A) or the second group (Group B); both groups contain equal calories. However, she is first invited outside for about an hour for a brisk walk, a short bike ride and some stretches and exercises in the garden, all of which use up about 600 calories. On her return, she showers and dresses, now pleasantly hungry and ready for the first meal of the day. Sitting down at the table, she surveys her meal choices, as follows:

Group A meals:

Breakfast Two poached eggs, one round of wholemeal toast, fresh fruit, tea or coffee	**Total calories**
Lunch Grilled fish with large salad, vinaigrette dressing, fresh fruit to follow	**2000**
Dinner Sirloin steak with field mushrooms, large side salad and steamed broccoli, one glass of Cabernet Sauvignon	

Group B meals:

Breakfast A two ounce slice of chocolate cake and large dollop of vanilla ice cream	
	Total calories
Lunch A two ounce slice of chocolate cake and large dollop of vanilla ice cream	**2000**
Dinner A two ounce slice of chocolate cake and large dollop of vanilla ice cream	

Will our volunteer lose weight on either meal group? Technically yes, as both meal plans contain 2000 calories, she will be in negative calorie balance to the tune of 600 calories on either Group (her BMR is 2000 calories plus 600 calories from exercise – 2000 calories from three meals today = minus 600 calories). Would she be hungry if she lived on Group B meals for any length of time? Yes. And would she be healthy if she lived on the Group B meals for weeks on end and nothing else? Err – no!

We can't live on chocolate cake alone

No one can live on portions of chocolate cake and ice cream for very long. Instead, let's consider two separate concepts in terms of weight loss and health. They are independent ideas but will need to be bundled up together into a holistic package of dietary and lifestyle changes by the time we are through. Let's think of becoming both slim and healthy using two headings (Fig 1):

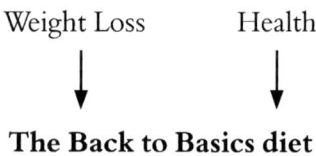

Fig 1: The holistic approach of the Back to Basics diet

Although some may argue this point, the vast majority of diets only address the issue of weight loss, i.e. calorie restriction. Some diets claim to do both but in reality, very few diets succeed in effectively combining calorie restriction *and* healthy eating over the long term. As we have seen in my somewhat flippant example, calorie restriction on its own is easy but we also need to address the *types* of food we eat as well. Losing weight whilst contracting scurvy is not the answer.

Calorie restriction, in isolation, is not enough

It is easy to design a diet that involves eating fewer calories – witness the chocolate cake and ice cream example. However, unless we reduce calories by eating the right sorts of foods, we are on a hiding to nothing. Living on tiny portions of modern, processed foods will never work – our genes are programmed to avoid starvation at all costs, so if we starve ourselves, our BMR will reduce and the hormonal signals that tell us to eat will start to bellow and we will fall off our diet. Guaranteed.

Living healthily, whilst steadily losing weight, is more important than jumping from one fad diet to another in the vain hope of a quick fix to our weight problems. That's why in Part 2 there is a sensible, real food-based weight loss plan, designed to reduce our calorie consumption naturally (with some simple new recipes), in combination with changes to when we eat our food during the day.

What's the big deal about losing weight?

Some people are genuinely happy to be overweight or obese. I have absolutely no problem with that at all but I suspect a doctor might take a different view. Unfortunately, carrying too much excess weight is likely to put us at risk of contracting numerous illnesses or even shorten our lives. For those who are thinking about trying to lose weight but are unhappy about the need to make fundamental changes to their diet or lifestyle, I offer this sobering thought:

If you or I continue to live as we are (i.e. eating the way we have always eaten and refraining from some sort of regular exercise), our obesity will simply get worse. We will remain on the obese person's 'conveyor belt of life', leading to something called metabolic syndrome, then pre-diabetes, then quite probably Type 2 diabetes, followed by all sorts of other nasty medical problems. Ultimately, we will be heading for an early grave.

I think we all deserve the chance to get off the conveyor belt. My hope is that by switching to a naturally low calorie, real food plant-based diet, we can reduce the chance of any health-related bad news at all. Unfortunately, our genes control us all, so some of us will be programmed for a difficult old age, whether we like it or not. Nevertheless, we can make a huge difference to our health and to the quality of our life by losing weight and getting to grips with a new, healthy lifestyle.

The Back to Basics diet is not a 'diet' at all

This book is not a diet as such (because diets don't work) but a structured programme to help re-establish a natural, healthy relationship with food. From now on, let's forget all about starvation, fad diets and tiny portions of chocolate cake – this is not the way to lose weight. Instead, by switching to a plant-based, real food diet, we can naturally reduce our calorie intake and lose weight, whilst giving ourselves a massive boost of healthy nutrients at the same time.

There is little doubt that our modern diet, full of sugar and artificial fats, is the root cause of the current obesity epidemic. Without giving us more than a smidgen of nutritional benefit, the highly processed foods that make up the bulk of our diet not only make us fat but also increase our risk of developing serious diseases. However, if we can grasp the nettle and strip the sugar and other processed foods from our diet, most of the causes of obesity will be removed in one fell swoop. By switching to an entirely real food diet, several issues resolve themselves straight away. We will automatically consume fewer calories. We will no longer try constantly to lay down fat for a rainy day and will recognize when we have eaten sufficient food. Finally, our cravings for sugar will ease and we will stabilize our blood sugar levels without having to eat something every five minutes.

Most of us are overweight because we have spent a lifetime eating the wrong sort of foods; not only have we consumed too many calories for little, if any, nutritional benefit, we have also sent our internal weight-regulating systems haywire, leading to steady and continual weight gain. Therefore, it is time to move away from fad and yo-yo dieting by embracing a new way of life, involving sensible, healthy eating and long-term weight loss, just as Nature intended.

It is time to eat the foods we are *designed* to eat, as we are about to find out.

3

Our hunter-gatherer origins

*Mankind differs from the animals only by a little
and most people throw that away.*
Confucius

To find out why our modern diet is so damaging to our health, we need to go back in time to find the original human diet. We can then start to unlock the dietary secrets that will rid us of our obesity and allow us to stay at our correct weight for the rest of our lives.

The original human diet can be traced back to Africa, where the earliest humans first appeared. These early humans (and *their* immediate ancestors) were hunter-gatherers who apparently lived healthy lives, free of most of our modern diseases. They paved the way for the much later appearance of what scientists call 'anatomically modern humans' a few hundred thousand years ago. In terms of what they needed to eat to keep them at the very peak of their powers, these early humans were identical to a much more modern version of a human known as you and me!

Evolution holds the key

The opening lecture of my biology degree began with a

PowerPoint slide containing the following quote:

*"Nothing in Biology Makes Sense Except in
the Light of Evolution"*
(Theodosius Dobzhansky; 1973)

As Charles Darwin discovered all those years ago, the process of evolution by natural selection underpins the entire natural world. Darwin worked with plants and animals but his ideas are equally relevant to our origins as human beings.

A very remarkable mammal

Millions of years of evolution, via natural selection, has led to a remarkably successful and intelligent mammal called a human being. We are truly amazing creatures, exquisitely designed by evolution and fine-tuned over millions of years to control our own weight. Today, many of us inadvertently abuse this wonderful body of ours by eating foods we are not designed to eat.[1] By delving into the story of human evolution, we begin to uncover the reasons why we put on weight so easily, why we are most certainly not adapted to our current diet and why the great scholar Professor Jared Diamond ('The Third Chimpanzee'; 'Guns, Germs and Steel' etc') described the invention of agriculture as "the worst mistake in the history of the human race".[2] By looking back at our earliest history on this planet and learning about the original human diet, we can start to make changes to *our* diet and lifestyle that will return us to a normal weight. In turn, this will help us live the longest and healthiest lives that our particular genetic throw of the dice will allow.

Our modern diet is making us ill

Our modern diet is so out of kilter with how we are designed to eat that we are literally poisoning ourselves with the foods we eat.[3] If we are to have any chance of finally getting to grips with our obesity, we need to understand why eating the way we do today is so at odds with how we are supposed to eat. To find out what we *should* be eating, we need to set off on a journey to our evolutionary past, back to the dawn of time when our ancestors, the early primates, ran wild and free across the Earth.

The story of 'us'

Our story begins about 65 million years ago (mya). This was when the earliest apes first started to appear in North America, before migrating to Africa to become the forerunner of all current living primates, including humans (see Fig 2).

We can trace our origins all the way back to these early apes. Our more recent ancestors developed from the earlier primates and appeared on Earth about 15mya. These very early prototype humans had large brains and were able to walk upright. However, it wasn't until much later (about 200,000 years ago) that we anatomically modern humans first made our entrance onto the stage of evolutionary history.[4] None of this happened overnight; it took millions of years

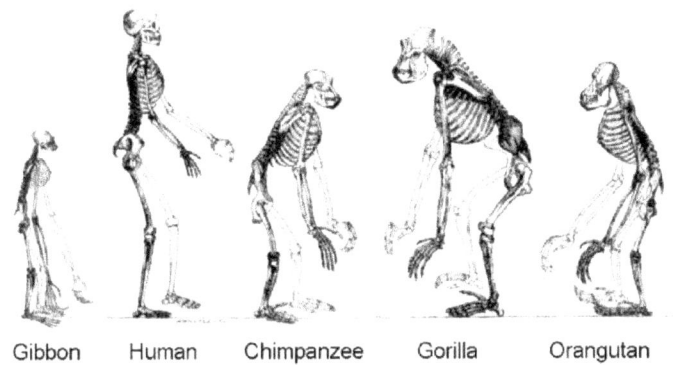

Gibbon   Human   Chimpanzee   Gorilla   Orangutan

Fig 2. The Third Chimpanzee? Our similarity to the Great Apes is clear from a comparison of primate skeletons (image courtesy of Wikipedia).

of evolution and natural selection before modern humans finally emerged on the scene, with many intermediate steps along the way.[5]

Australopithecus – our (very) early ancestors

One of the first prototype human groups ('genus' in science speak) was called *Australopithecus*.[6] The australopiths had brains about 35% the size of ours and stood just 4 feet tall but were quite a successful bunch. They walked upright, the first evidence of bi-pedalism in our ancestry. No one is quite sure why we started walking on our hind legs but the academics are convinced this ability to walk upright probably played a major role in the later development of our large human brains.

THE STORY OF US

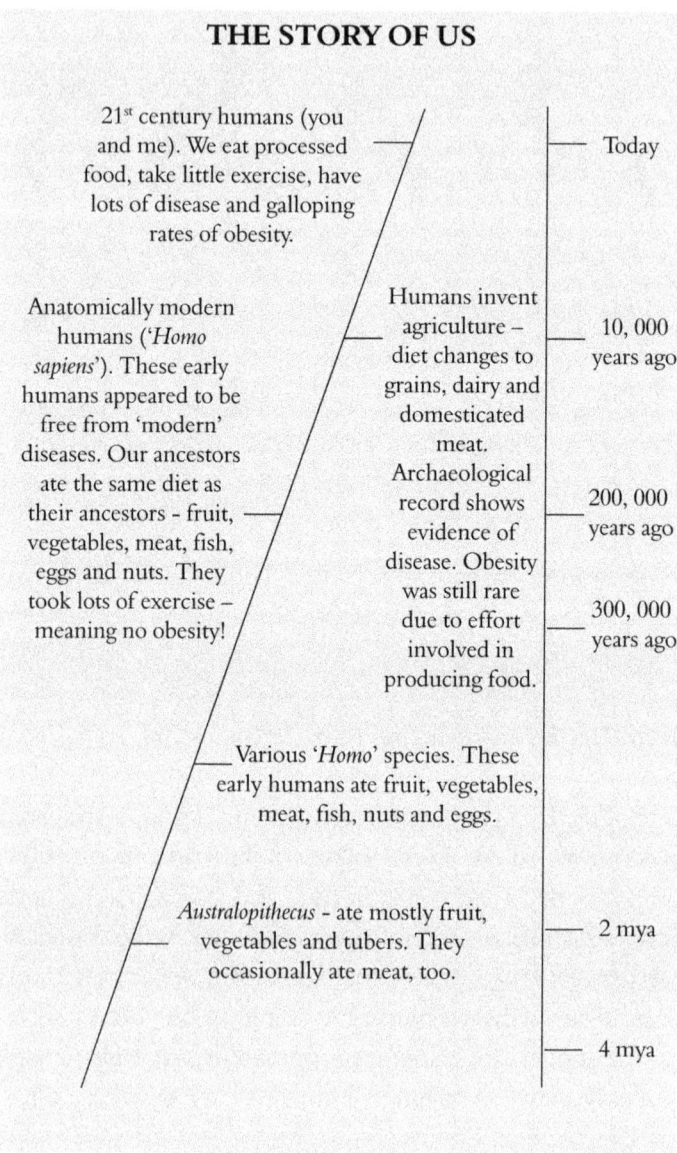

21ˢᵗ century humans (you and me). We eat processed food, take little exercise, have lots of disease and galloping rates of obesity.

Anatomically modern humans ('*Homo sapiens*'). These early humans appeared to be free from 'modern' diseases. Our ancestors ate the same diet as their ancestors - fruit, vegetables, meat, fish, eggs and nuts. They took lots of exercise – meaning no obesity!

Humans invent agriculture – diet changes to grains, dairy and domesticated meat. Archaeological record shows evidence of disease. Obesity was still rare due to effort involved in producing food.

Various '*Homo*' species. These early humans ate fruit, vegetables, meat, fish, nuts and eggs.

Australopithecus - ate mostly fruit, vegetables and tubers. They occasionally ate meat, too.

Today

10, 000 years ago

200, 000 years ago

300, 000 years ago

2 mya

4 mya

26

The original Back to Basics diet

So, what did the australopiths eat? By looking at the patterns of wear on australopith fossil teeth, scientists have worked out that our earliest ancestors ate a diet almost exclusively consisting of fruit, vegetables and tubers; some of the more robust *Australopithecus* species also ate nuts and seeds. A few ate the odd lizard, too.

Australopithecus probably died out about 2mya. Not all living creatures prove successful in the long term – that's evolution for you. The next prototype humans to appear were species of the genus *Homo*. Today, humans ('*Homo sapiens*') are the last surviving species of this genus but in the past there were a number of *Homo* species, some of which were directly involved in the development of modern humans.

Out of Africa

There are essentially two different theories as to what happened next; either we modern humans evolved separately back in Africa[7] (about 250,000 years ago) and then spread out to replace all the original *Homo* populations or we arose independently from various earlier *Homo* populations already spread across the globe.[8,9] Regardless of which theory is correct, anatomically modern humans, pretty much the same as you and me, appeared on Planet Earth about 200,000 years ago.

It seems the early *Homo* species ate what the australopiths ate but supplemented their diet with meat and fish.[10] This diet appears to have kept our earliest ancestors fit and healthy; as far as I am aware, no significant evidence of heart disease or cancers has yet been found in the archaeology of these early humans.[11]

The hunter-gatherer diet

Although we evolved from a plant-eating ancestor, at some point our ancestors must have started to eat meat. This was regarded as a relatively recent change to human dietary patterns until the discovery of 'Lucy', the skeleton of an early species of *Australopithecus* in Ethiopia in 1974. Lucy was about 3.2 million years old and appeared to have used stone tools to cut the meat off animal bones, presumably for her dinner. It seems we became carnivores much earlier than first thought.[12]

Until the advent of agriculture, about 10,000 years ago (less than the blink of an eye in evolutionary terms), all humans evolved on a diet of basically the same food. Regardless of when we started to eat meat, there were no shops, no takeaways and no restaurants, so all food was wild and had to be gathered (wild fruits and vegetables) or hunted or scavenged. The specifics varied across the globe but many features of the ancestral diet were remarkably consistent:

- No processed food
- Not much grain
- No dairy and virtually no sugar
- No modern 'man-made' fats

The secret to the perfect diet is in the shape of our gut

We share about 98.4% of our DNA with chimpanzees, so it should be no surprise to discover that humans and chimpanzees are designed to eat a very similar diet. The good news, however, is that we are not designed to eat the *same* diet as a chimpanzee.

Everything hinges on the size and shape of our colon! Both humans and chimps have a 'sacculated' or 'haustrated' colon, a sure sign that we are derived from a plant-eating ancestor.[13] Similarly, neither humans nor chimps can synthesize Vitamin C, which is best obtained from fruits and vegetables in the diet. These aspects of our digestion (plus the shape of our teeth) confirm that we are descended from a plant-eating ancestor.

Fortunately, humans are *not* chimpanzees

Chimps have much bigger colons than we do, whereas we have more of our gut as small intestine. This makes a big difference to our respective diets; chimps have to eat loads of tough plant material to obtain their nutrition (which is then broken down slowly by fermentation in their huge colons), whilst humans have become adapted to a high-quality diet of fruits, vegetables and animal foods,[14] which better suits our digestive design. Both apes and humans are unusual in the time it takes for food to transit through the body compared to a carnivore (it takes roughly 45 hours for high-fibre food to transit our guts, whereas a polar bear will poop out the remains of his seal dinner in about 17 hours). This is important for weight loss, as we will see later.

THE DESIGN OF OUR GUT SHOWS US THE WAY TO OUR PERFECT DIET

- The shape of our intestines means we are descended from a plant-eating ancestor; we are designed to eat fruits and vegetables.
- We can't make Vitamin C, so we are supposed to get this micronutrient from the fruit and vegetables in our diet.
- The differences in our gut design compared to chimps' shows that we are meant to eat a high-quality diet of fruit and vegetables, 'topped off' with meats and fish.
- Our guts have a limited capacity because we are designed to eat a predominantly vegetarian diet. This means we are supposed to fill up with healthy, low-calorie, nutrient-rich plant food which takes a while to digest and so stops us from otherwise eating too many calories (from junk food?). Add some legumes, a few nuts, and some (organic) meat or fish to our diet and we end up very close to the diet that evolution has spent millions of years perfecting.

Our recent ancestors ate a perfect diet, too

Wild chimpanzees don't seem to suffer from obesity or modern diseases and neither did our ancient ancestors, as far as we can tell from the archaeological record. We also find very low rates of obesity and modern diseases in many contemporary hunter-gatherer societies and in people who until recently maintained a traditional lifestyle, e.g. subsistence farmers in Crete up to the 1970s.[15,16]

What can we learn from these remarkable people? Well, they took a lot of exercise and so used up a lot of calories every day. They ate food that was naturally low in calories but high in nutrients, i.e. a mostly vegetarian diet, with meat or fish on high days and holidays. The key here is "mostly vegetarian" – just like our ancestors, the original human hunter-gatherer diet was predominantly vegetarian, with opportunistic meat eating now and again as hunting is actually quite difficult and often unsuccessful. And due to the slow passage of food through the human gut, our ancestors could fill up on plant food (so meeting their needs for energy) and make use of infrequent meals of animal protein and fats to add high-quality nutrients to their diet. This is much more efficient than your average chimp who has to eat vastly more plant food in order to gain a complete array of nutrients.

Agriculture – the biggest mistake in human history?

Unfortunately, everything went a bit south about 10,000 years ago when the human race invented agriculture. At first glance, this seems like a huge leap forward in the evolution of Man, as for first time food availability could be pretty much guaranteed. By growing crops and raising livestock, these early farmers were able to break the seasonal cycle of feast or famine common to all hunter-gatherer societies.

However, the skeletal remains of the early agriculturists appear to be shorter, misshapen with disease and obviously much less healthy than skeletons found in the fossil record from any number of earlier hunter-gatherer communities.[17] Perhaps this was why Jared Diamond called the invention of agriculture "the biggest mistake in human history"? To be fair, he was talking mostly about sociological issues but something obviously went badly awry with the human diet when, as a species, we decided to abandon our evolutionary past as hunters and adopt the plough instead. Ironically, the problem stems from something to do with plants.

Plants want to survive, too

Plants have been around a long time and although they appear at first glance to be less sophisticated than animals and humans, the pressures of natural selection have led to remarkable strategies in plants to help them successfully pass on their genes.[18]

Plants have a tough life – they have to compete with their neighbours for nutrients and water from the soil and have to fight for access to sunlight, so they can grow and store energy through photosynthesis. Meanwhile, they have to deal with passing animals that take great delight in eating their leaves and stems for lunch. Plants pass on their genes through their seeds, which contain the genetic information ready for the next generation. Many plants encase their seeds in highly nutritious and colourful fruits, which they are more than happy for the passing mammal to eat. This way, the seeds pass through the digestive tract of the animal in question and are deposited somewhere else in the forest, so spreading the genes of this particular plant species far and wide – evolution in action. However, the plant does *not* want its seeds eaten and destroyed. Consequently, many plants have evolved numerous cunning ways to make their seeds unpalatable (or often, downright poisonous) to animal grazers. As an example, let's look at a fairly well known plant called wheat.

Why eating wheat is generally not a good idea

Eating our daily bread is an integral part of life, the food that defines us as a civilized society. Bread is mostly made from wheat, the wheat grain being ground to make flour, which is then used to make bread and lots of other gooey, sticky delights. Technically, a wheat grain is a combination of a fruit and a seed but we can just think of the grain of wheat as wheat seed. Wheat grains have been at the heart of the Western diet for thousands of years, proving to be a nutritious food source from the very earliest days of agriculture. However, is wheat grain a natural human food?

Gluten and lectin – two reasons to give wheat a wide berth

The wheat seed contains substances that turn out to be rather nasty when consumed by humans.[19] Gluten is used by grass-type plants, like wheat, as a food source in the seed for the new plant embryo during germination. Lectins are proteins

THE PROBLEM OF WHEAT

- We eat the seeds of the wheat plant in the form of flour.
- Like all plants, wheat wants to protect its seeds at all costs.
- The wheat plant has evolved some unpleasant chemicals (particularly gluten and lectin) that are mainly designed to do other tasks but happen to make the seeds of the wheat plant unpalatable.
- The chemicals in the seeds of a wheat plant means that wheat flour is most definitely not a natural human food.
- Processed ('white') bread provides too many calories for only a modicum of nutrition, is directly linked to the causes of obesity and can lead to potentially life-threatening illness and disease.
- Fancy that sandwich now?

that can bind to various sugars in cells and then help out with lots of complex cellular tasks. So these two substances, gluten and lectin, are designed by evolution to help wheat–type plants (rye, barley etc) pass on their genes. However, that doesn't mean that we are designed to eat wheat seeds ourselves.

Gluten and lectin are proteins, so must provide us with some of our daily protein requirement? Yes and no. Yes, they provide us with a source of protein but they also make us ill and are now known to be a major contributor to the obesity epidemic we see all around us.

GLUTEN AND LECTIN

*(Some very good reasons why we should give
wheat a wide berth)*

- Gluten (and one of its proteins called *gliadin*) causes inflammation of the gut in most people. It is believed that coeliac disease, a serious autoimmune condition, is caused by the body's intolerance to the gliadin protein in gluten.
- Most of us are intolerant to the effects of gluten in our diet. This leads to inflammation of the gut ('leaky gut'), where chemicals that should remain in the gut, such as the toxins from nasty bacteria, can cross into the blood stream and do damage around the body.
- Such inflammation and leaky gut means our immune system makes antibodies, which can then cause untold problems elsewhere. Gliadin has a similar chemical structure to proteins in other parts of our body (e.g. in the thyroid and the pancreas), so the antibodies end up attacking these other proteins 'by mistake'!
- There is also evidence that antibodies to gluten might be implicated in both heart disease and cancer, too.
- Lectin also upsets our guts, causing inflammation and leaky gut. In terms of obesity, lectin interferes with a chemical signaling system in the body that is designed to tell us we are full, so stop eating! If these signals are ignored, we don't realize we are full and keep eating! Result – we eat too many calories and get fat.

Our hunter-gatherer ancestors point the way to a perfect diet

For much of human history, mankind existed in tribes and communities around the world that lived in a similar way.[20] Even though the content of the diet varied due to geography, all foods eaten prior to the invention of agriculture were real, unprocessed foods (vegetables, fruit, meat, naturally-occurring fats, poultry, fish, nuts, eggs etc). By happy coincidence, such unprocessed food is fairly low in calories, too. Unprocessed food does not, generally, lead to inflammation in the body. Unprocessed food is full of natural, healthy proteins, fats and healthy carbohydrates plus abundant micronutrients, such as minerals, vitamins and the catch-all 'phytonutrients', the wonderful life-giving and irreplaceable chemicals found in fruits and vegetables. As a species we are *not* designed to live almost exclusively on the seeds of four plants, i.e. wheat, rice, corn and rye.

It is time to wave goodbye to 'baked goods'

If we are determined to lose weight effectively and avoid numerous medical problems that stem from a leaky gut then we would all be better off giving bread, cakes and other baked goods the old heave-ho and embracing a predominantly plant-based diet instead. This allows us to plan our meals around plant food that is relatively low in calories but rich in nutrients, i.e. full of all the vitamins, anti-oxidants, proteins, healthy fats etc essential for health.

For even the most dedicated carnivores, this is not as bad as it sounds. A 'predominantly plant-based diet' still means we can enjoy our Sunday lunch, steaks, roast chicken, fresh fish, pork chops etc – it just means we are going to replace all the processed foods in our diet with fresh fruits, salads and vegetables and combine them with tasty sources of animal protein. And by filling up on veggies, we won't need much meat, poultry, or fish anyway, so will almost certainly spend less money than we used to spend on processed junk back in the old days. By adding some legumes, a few nuts and seeds and some organic meat or fish to our plant-based diet, we end up eating in accord with our evolutionary design and in a way that has enabled millions of people across the globe to avoid obesity and enjoy a healthy, happy life.

Add some onions and garlic, a little olive oil, the odd glass of red wine and the company of good friends and family and we arrive at my favourite version of Back to Basics eating, a traditional (and fairly low-carbohydrate) Mediterranean diet. Naturally low in calories and bursting with healthy nutrients, a Back to Basics Mediterranean diet is one of the best ways to eat for both weight loss and health and I heartily recommend it to those who enjoy such flavours of the sun.

It is time to enjoy real food again and to buy and cook seasonal fruits and vegetables and source healthy, organic sources of protein. From now on, I hope we can all forget about fad diets and yo-yo dieting and instead look forward to a new way of life, involving sensible, healthy eating and long-term weight loss.

Let's now turn to food itself; what it comprises, what it is made of and why some knowledge of food science will help us understand why our modern diet is so alien to the way we are designed to eat.

4

The food we eat

*'I do not like broccoli. And I haven't liked it since I was
a little kid and my mother made me eat it. And I'm President
of the United States and I'm not going to eat any more broccoli.'*
President George Bush

Food – friend and foe?

Real food is key to permanent weight loss and much
improved health but we live in a world where such food can
be quite hard to find. Instead, high-calorie, processed foods
exist everywhere we look.[1] Nevertheless, to lose weight
effectively and keep that weight off for life, we know we need
to make a clean break from such unhealthy foods in favour of
a more traditional, natural and sustainable diet. We will cover
'real food' in detail later but first, let's have a brief look at the
components of our diet and see how we can make better food
choices in future.

The chemistry of life

Our bodies are extraordinarily complex and contain a
baffling array of cells, tissues and organs. Literally millions of

chemical reactions take place inside these cells and organs all the time, each one of which allows us to live, grow and exist as a healthy human being. These chemical reactions are usually referred to as human biochemistry, meaning the 'chemistry of life'; how all these biochemical reactions interplay to make us work is referred to as human physiology. We don't need any more detail than that but you might see me refer to these terms in later chapters.

Metabolism

When we eat something, the various foodstuffs are broken down in our digestive system to their component parts. This breaking down process, known as *catabolism*, is how we obtain the building blocks for all the other chemicals and substances we have to make to keep us alive. This is one part of our overall metabolism. During catabolism, energy is released as something called ATP (effectively the petrol of our body chemistry 'engine'). Later, we use these building blocks in a complementary process called *anabolism*, where new chemicals and products are built up from scratch, using the energy of ATP, as previously released during catabolism.

You may have heard of the drugs used by some misguided athletes known as anabolic steroids? These drugs are designed to enhance anabolism or build up of cells, particularly in muscles, of course.

So, there are two distinct processes (catabolism and anabolism) that occur during and after eating food. Much

METABOLISM – THE TECHNICAL STUFF

- Metabolism is the sum of all the biochemical processes in our bodies that allow us to function as a healthy human being. There are a vast number of chemical reactions involved in metabolism but in terms of our weight, there are two key processes, known as *catabolism* and *anabolism*.
- Catabolism is the breaking down of big molecules into smaller bits, during which energy is released. Catabolism can either be the breakdown of the foods we eat at each meal or the 'burning' of stored food (e.g. glycogen, fat) to use in lieu of food. The process of catabolism releases energy in the form of ATP, to drive our body chemistry. Catabolism is controlled by numerous hormones, e.g. cortisol, glucagon, adrenalin.
- Anabolism is the opposite of catabolism and involves the building up of complex molecules from smaller bits (e.g. new cells and tissue, such as muscle). Anabolism requires energy (ATP) and is mediated by hormones too, e.g. the anabolic steroids and insulin.
- If catabolism exceeds anabolism, there will be an excess of energy. We store this excess as either glycogen or fat.
- So, our body weight = catabolism *minus* anabolism. To *lose weight*, anabolism needs to *exceed* catabolism (i.e. by eating fewer calories).

of the reason we put on weight is due to imbalances in these two biochemical systems, simply because our present way of eating is out of balance with our biochemistry.[2]

The components of our diet

Scientists generally talk about food under one of two main headings; *macro*nutrients make up the bulk of the food we eat, whilst *micro*nutrients are the invisible components of our diet that are responsible for boosting our health and fighting disease (Fig 3):

MACRONUTRIENTS	MICRONUTRIENTS
Protein	Water
Fat (triglycerides)	Vitamins
Carbohydrates	Minerals Anti-oxidants Phytochemicals etc

Fig 3. The classification of foods by nutrient content

I think it is much more useful to think about food being either 'real' or 'processed'. This makes it much easier to make healthy choices when we are shopping or when eating out in restaurants etc. However, for now I will stick with the official system. In many ways, it is the amount of micronutrients in our diet that decides our level of health and wellbeing but here I want to concentrate on the main classes of food that we have all heard of, namely, the macronutrients:

Protein

Proteins are long–chain molecules made up from linked subunits called amino acids. Amino acids can be linked up in longer and longer chains to form protein molecules. Of the 22 amino acids known to exist, nine are classed as essential; this means we are unable to make these particular amino acids ourselves and so have to take them in through our diet to maintain our health.[3]

Amino acids	
Essential amino acids	**Non-essential amino acids**
Histidine	Alanine
Isoleucine	Arginine
Leucine	Asparagine
Lysine	Aspartic acid
Methionine	Cysteine
Phenylalanine	Glutamic acid
Threonine	Glycine
Tryptophan	Ornithine
Valine	Proline
	Selenocysteine
	Serine
	Taurine
	Tyrosine

As most of the important processes in our bodies rely on protein in one form or another, proteins are obviously vital to our health. The growth and renewal of our cells and organs depends on the presence of proteins, whilst virtually every chemical reaction that takes place inside us is controlled by a protein known as an enzyme, a catalyst that speeds up chemical reactions.[4] Proteins are involved in myriad other biological tasks as well. However, there is one group of proteins that we have touched on already that are at the heart of the obesity/weight loss story; these crucial proteins are called hormones and we will meet some of them again later.

Thinking about protein conjures up images of large steaks sizzling on the barbeque but it is largely a myth that we have to eat lots of animal food to get our daily protein requirements. We can easily get all the protein we need from plants, e.g. fruit, vegetables, nuts, seeds, legumes etc.[5] However, unless you are barred from such foods on religious, ethical or moral grounds, it is easier to put together a healthy, effective weight loss diet by including small amounts of natural (ideally organic) animal foods, such as fish and small amounts of unprocessed meats. We'll talk about proteins again later on, so for now let's look at the other classes of macronutrients.

Fats – a 'potted' history

I believe there is a fundamental misunderstanding about the role of fat in a healthy diet, so here is a quick run through of fats in a bit more detail.[6]

Ancel Keys

Up until about the time of the Second World War, the most common medical treatment for obesity was a low carbohydrate diet, i.e. eat meat and fats but avoid the carbs. This all goes back to the Victorian era, when a rather corpulent Englishman called William Banting famously made public the story of his weight loss on just such a diet (an interesting story; for more details see Gary Taubes's book 'Good Calories, Bad Calories').[7]

However, after the War an American scientist named Ancel Keys claimed that high levels of saturated fat in the diet led to heart disease. Although nothing to do with obesity, this hypothesis was seized upon as gospel by the US Government, which later published the famous 'eat a low fat, high carbohydrate diet for health' mantra, advice that has dominated the world of human nutrition for the last fifty years.[8,9]

Regardless of the history, to many of us who are trying to lose weight, fat is a dirty word, so what is the latest thinking on fat in our diet?

Both the fats in our diet and the fat we carry around our bodies are known as triglycerides. A triglyceride is a molecule that consists of a backbone of an alcohol called glycerol attached to three (hence 'tri') fatty acids (see Fig 4).

The Cs and Hs are just chemistry short hand for many atoms of carbon (the C), joined to many atoms of hydrogen (the H). Carbon needs to form four chemical bonds to be stable electrically, so if each carbon atom in the fatty acid chain makes all four bonds, our fat is *saturated*, i.e. all the bonds of each carbon atom are complete. However, if there isn't enough hydrogen to go round, carbon can be crafty and form a double bond with an adjacent carbon atom instead, so

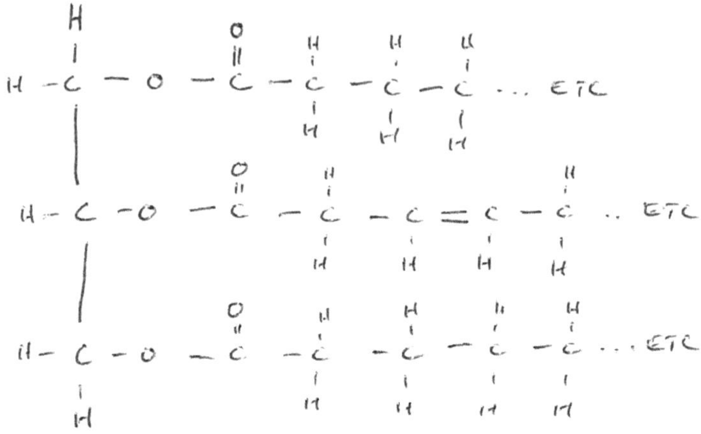

Fig 4. The component parts of a triglyceride

making an *unsaturated* fat. If just one double bond is formed, the fat is said to be a 'mono'-unsaturated, fat e.g. olive oil. If there is more than one double bond in the fatty acid chain, then the fat is referred to as 'poly'-unsaturated, e.g. numerous vegetable oils.

The energy in fats

Fat is a very efficient source of energy; if you burned some in a laboratory, it would yield nine calories of heat energy per gram of weight. This is compared to most carbohydrates (i.e. sugars) that only yield four calories of heat energy per gram. Fat, therefore, is an excellent source of energy. Saturated fats such as butter and lard are usually solids at room temperatures because of the bulky three-dimensional molecular shape needed to cram in all those hydrogen atoms. Mono- and poly-unsaturated fats are generally liquid at room temperatures.

Getting our 'Omegas' in the right proportion

Similar to the essential amino acids in proteins, there are also essential fatty acids that we have to obtain through our diet. These fatty acids are vital to our health (they are used, amongst other things, to build our cell walls and manufacture hormones) and act as the building blocks of other fatty acids that we can make ourselves.[10]

The two main essential fatty acids are called linoleic acid, an Omega 6 fatty acid, and alpha-linolenic acid, an Omega 3 fatty acid (the '6' and the '3' just refer to the position of the double bond in the fatty acid chain). One of the most important aspects of a healthy diet is getting these two fatty acids in the right proportion.[11]

We evolved to eat Omega 3 and Omega 6 fatty acids in a ratio close to one to one or thereabouts.[12] This was relatively easy for our stone age ancestors because the real, natural foods they ate had a balance of Omega 6 : Omega 3 in the correct ratio. However, most modern, processed foods contain far too much Omega 6 but not enough Omega 3, completely upsetting that natural balance.

Modern, processed foods are known to cause inflammation in our bodies, which is a similar reaction to the one our immune system mounts when we injure ourselves, for instance. Such internal inflammation can lead to numerous chronic diseases, such as heart disease and increased risk of cancer, but is also directly related to obesity and modern 'diseases of civilization', including Type 2 diabetes.[13]

Sugar is one of the leading culprits behind this immune response but inflammation is also caused by an Omega 6 fatty acid called arachidonic acid. This particular Omega 6 fatty acid raises the level of the hormone insulin, which, as we will see later, causes untold problems, too. However, if we eat sufficient quantities of Omega 3 in our diet, we increase the level of another type of Omega 3 fatty acid called DHA which has powerful anti-inflammatory effects. Unfortunately, most of us eat a diet that is way too high in Omega 6 fats and correspondingly too low in Omega 3 fats, which contributes to the internal inflammation that is so damaging to our health.

Omega 3 is found in certain plants (such as flaxseed) and also in many oily fish, e.g. mackerel, tuna, sardines. To strike the correct balance between the Omega 6 fats and the Omega 3 fats in our diet, we need to bin most of the sources of Omega 6 fats (largely found in many processed foods) and eat more Omega 3 foods.

Trans fats – the real fat enemy

Along with too much sugar, 'trans' fats are a major cause of the obesity epidemic and associated ill health seen today all around the world.[14,15] Sometimes referred to as 'hydrogenated' fats, these are fats that are not natural in nature but are instead manufactured by the food industry to extend the shelf life of processed foods. Natural poly-unsaturated and mono-unsaturated fats are changed by hydrogen-ation, i.e. the artificial addition of hydrogen atoms to break the double bonds in the fatty acid chains, thereby creating a man-made saturated fat. This gives big profits to the food industry as such fats can resist oxidation (going rancid) for much longer than a natural fat. All in all, these fats are bad news and should be avoided as much as possible.

Saturated fats

Since writing the first edition of the book, my views on saturated fats have changed somewhat, so what follows here is my latest thinking on these rather infamous fats.

Saturated fats have always been part of the human diet, being hugely important in the diet of our ancestors and often the main source of calories and nutrients for aboriginal peoples such as the Inuit and certain Plains Native Americans.[16] Saturated fats do contain numerous helpful vitamins and are a highly efficient source of energy.[17] And yes, if saturated fat was inherently toxic, millions of years of evolution and natural selection would have come up with a different way of storing energy inside our bodies. So, in many ways, real, unprocessed fat is a perfectly natural human food.[18,19] I certainly have no objection to fats, saturated or otherwise, that occur naturally in plants or in fresh, unprocessed poultry and fish. However, I now try to reduce my consumption of most saturated fats (fatty meats, butter, some cheeses etc), preferring to replace them with plant foods, some fish, fruits and a little olive oil now and again.

Fats – drawing a line in the sand

There is a constant to and fro in the scientific literature between those who believe we should eat unrestricted amounts of fat but avoid the carbs and those to whom even a teaspoon of olive oil is tantamount to immediate cardiac failure[20–28]. This is at best confusing and at worst totally unhelpful when we are trying to decide what to eat so we can lose weight and improve our health. After much reading of the recent literature and subsequent head scratching, I have come to the opinion that *adding* fats to our plant-based, real food diet (in the form of butter, animal fats, excessive amounts of olive oil etc) is probably not a good idea. I am not alone; the American Heart Association recently reduced the recommended level of saturated fat in the diet to just 5% of total food intake. The whole subject of carbs can be equally confusing, as we will see in a moment but simply replacing carbohydrate foods with fat and hoping for the best is not a sensible way to construct a healthy, lifelong eating plan. I would not worry unduly about the fat content of fish or lean, organic meats and poultry but recommend obtaining most of our fats from unprocessed plant foods that contain natural fats, such as olives and avocados. In terms of added fats, my preference now is for virgin olive oil and only in small amounts.

Carbohydrates

Carbohydrates or carbs feature high up the list of any discussion about calories, weight loss or which diet to follow. Carbs dominate many modern diets – the 'high-carb, low fat' diet, the 'low carb' diet, the 'low carb, high fat' diet etc. No wonder we are so confused about what to eat. Nevertheless, I firmly believe that the root cause of the obesity epidemic is the availability of heavily processed, highly calorific carbohydrate foods everywhere we look. *Processed* carbs are plant foods that have been changed in some way in a factory, e.g. wheat turned into flour into bread. Carbs are obviously an important part of our story, so let's take a closer look at this rather infamous foodstuff.

Carbohydrates are made from sugar

Carbohydrates are the sugars and starches we all love to hate. Most carbs are built up from small molecules called monosaccharides (i.e. glucose, fructose and galactose), which form the building blocks of more complex carbohydrates. Next up are the disaccharides (such as sucrose or 'table sugar'), which is made from glucose and fructose and then on pretty much ad infinitum to something called a polysaccharide. Most carbohydrates are made by one of Nature's more amazing chemical processes called photosynthesis. Photosynthesis, fundamental to life on Earth, takes place in the green parts of plants. Here, light energy from the Sun is used to combine carbon dioxide from the atmosphere with water to make carbohydrate (glucose) and oxygen:

**PHOTOSYNTHESIS
(THE KEY TO LIFE ON EARTH)**
(light energy from the Sun)
carbon dioxide + water = **carbohydrate (glucose)**
+ oxygen

Much of the food we are designed to eat contains carbohydrate, e.g. fruits and vegetables. However, many of the foods we live on today are made from processed carbohydrate and as we shall see, it is these foods that cause us problems. Such processed carbohydrate foods include bread, pastries, pasta, white rice, sweets, soft drinks, beer, fried potatoes, cakes, chocolates etc. The crux of the matter is that carbohydrates are made from sugar. This includes foods that appear savoury to our taste, e.g. white bread, pasta, white rice. Carbohydrates in their natural form are a vital part of the human diet but things start to go belly up when we humans (aka the food industry) start messing around with carbohydrates in an attempt to mass produce cheap, easily distributed food. Unfortunately, such processed carbs are everywhere and make up the bulk of many people's diets, often with disastrous consequences.[29,30]

Starch

Plants store energy in the form of starch, a polysaccharide made from glucose molecules linked together by chemical bonds. Starch is found in abundance in foods such as potatoes and grains, e.g. wheat. When we eat starch, the large starch molecule is broken down to glucose by our digestive system, leading to lots of glucose molecules entering the blood stream. Glucose is an important foodstuff (and the main 'food' for our brains) but the digestion of starch can be a double-edged sword, as too much glucose in the bloodstream will cause us problems, as we will see later.

Sugar – probably the root cause of our obesity

Carbohydrates are made of sugar but healthy foods such as fruits and vegetables also contain carbohydrate and hence sugar, too. However, when I talk about 'sugar', I am specifically talking about the sugar in modern, processed foods, the foods many of us eat every day. So, let's deal with the whole question of sugar and find out why a high sugar diet is just about the worst diet we could ever eat.[31]

When I first read the book *Eat to Live* by Dr Joel Fuhrman,[32] I was struck by his explanation of how our health is governed by the ratio of calories to nutrients in our diet. I call this the "Fuhrman Equation" as it is such a clever and succinct way of summing up how we should eat. In a nutshell, the Fuhrman Equation is this:

$$\text{'Health'} = \text{Nutrients}/\text{Calories}$$
or in algebraic terms, $\text{'}H\text{'} = N/C$

In other words, our health is governed by the ratio of nutrients to calories in our diet, with the best health score derived from a diet that is very high in nutrients but correspondingly low in calories. Where does sugar fit into this scenario? Well, many experts describe sugar as an 'anti-nutrient', for the simple fact that sugar supplies excessive calories for essentially no nutritional benefit. Yes, sugar supplies calories but it is not really a natural part of the human diet – early wild fruits were not terribly sweet. Some sugars are basically toxins, much like alcohol and recreational drugs.

SUGAR

- Sugar supplies excess calories for little nutritional benefit.
- Excess sugar consumption (mostly in the form of processed carbohydrate) is directly linked to obesity.
- Sugar consumption is a major contributing factor to Type 2 diabetes.
- Sugar is implicated in a number of cancers, including breast, colon and stomach cancer.
- Sugar is very addictive – the food industry knows this!
- To re-establish a healthy relationship with food and lose weight, most sugar (some fruit is OK) needs to be stripped from the diet.

There is very good evidence that excess sugar consumption not only leads to obesity but is a major contributory factor in Type 2 diabetes and heart disease.[33] Even more disturbing is the suggestion that sugar is implicated in a number of cancers, including breast, colon and stomach cancer. The two key dietary sugars are glucose and fructose (see box). Much of the reason we get so fat today is because of very high levels of these sugars in our modern diet.

It's time to 'let go' of sugar

Dietary processed sugar is so far away from what we should be eating that we need to bid it a fond farewell, once and for all. Sugar is very addictive so this won't be easy but if we can stick with it, we will be empowered to make a massive, positive difference to our lives and give ourselves the best chance of success with this or any other sensible diet and lifestyle programme. Giving up sugar is a big step for many of us but one that will make a huge difference to our ability to take back control of our weight and long-term health, once and for all.

The Glycaemic Index

Real, natural plant foods (containing carbohydrate) should make up the bulk of our diet but many of us are overweight because our diet contains far too many carbs. Much of this confusion can be laid to rest by looking at the Glycaemic Index (GI), a system for categorizing the carbohydrates in our diet.

The GI ranks carbohydrate foods against a reference of glucose in terms of how quickly the carbohydrate food in question raises our blood sugar level.[34,35] Glucose is given a value of 100 on the Index, whilst the lowest point

GLUCOSE AND FRUCTOSE
(TWO KEY SUGARS)

- Glucose is a natural human food source and the end product of most carbohydrate digestion. Glucose is the fuel of choice for important organs such as the brain, kidneys and red blood cells. However, excess glucose in the bloodstream can lead directly to obesity.

- Fructose is found in small quantities in fruit but most fructose is eaten as part of sucrose (table sugar). There has been a huge increase in fructose consumption since the 1960s (especially in the US), due to the invention of High Fructose Corn Syrup (HFCS), a cheap, easily mass-produced source of sugar. Unlike glucose, which has an important dietary role, fructose is treated by our metabolism much like alcohol, a known toxin. Like alcohol, fructose is processed exclusively in the liver where it is converted to *fat*.

on the index is zero, i.e. no effect on blood sugar levels at all. Foods containing carbohydrates are ranked against glucose; the idea is that glucose is glucose, so obviously is 'top of the charts' in terms of affecting the corresponding blood glucose concentration. Foods high on the index cause rapid increases in blood glucose levels, whilst foods low on the index show a much slower (or lesser) blood glucose response.

Most foods that are low on the index (which is good) are

fruits, vegetables, some legumes and grains in their natural state. Most of the foods high on the index are processed carbohydrates, e.g. white bread, chips, cornflakes, ice cream, tomato ketchup. The GI is not perfect but if we eat low on the index, much of the confusion about which carbs we should eat is resolved. Nevertheless, this is largely academic, as the recommended foods of the Back to Basics diet are all naturally very low on the GI, so no need to refer back to the Index in the future.

By the way, there are no such things as essential carbohydrates and we could, in theory, live perfectly happily in a carbohydrate-free world. However, the Back to Basics diet is most definitely not a carb-free diet.[22] We will talk more about how carbs fit into our new, healthy diet at some length later in the book.

So, what are we going to eat?

Let's move on from the food science now and focus instead on all the wonderful foods we can eat on the Back to Basics programme. These are nutritious, tasty, natural foods that are going to form the basis of our diet in the future, foods that are relatively cheap to buy, abundantly available and able to be made into a huge variety of delicious meals. Hopefully they will prove to be a delight to eat as well.

Sticking to local foods

The Back to Basics diet does not require any obscure or

weird ingredients – you know the ones, found growing on a rare tree in the Himalayas and picked at dawn by a virgin on a Tuesday when the moon is full? OK, I am being silly, but many fad diets expect us to search out the most bizarre and obscure foods imaginable. This is yet another reason why many diets fail in the long term, so everything that follows here is about learning to seek out and choose the right foods, whether from our local shops and supermarkets or when eating out in pubs and restaurants etc.

No specialist cooking skills required

There is no need to spend all day in the kitchen preparing complicated meals on the Back to Basics programme. Later, I will introduce some simple meal ideas, made from real, tasty food, which you can prepare in double-quick time. This means you don't have to spend hours toiling away in the kitchen where temptation lies in wait. However, if you love cooking and feel that it would help you come to terms with your new diet by playing around with recipes and creating more elaborate meals, then please be my guest.

The foods of the Back to Basics diet

Let's now look at all the wonderful foods that are going to form the basis of the Back to Basics diet. I will consider each food category from a UK shopping and home cook perspective but the basic principles apply to all of us, regardless of where we live.

Good carbs – fruit and vegetables

Many of us have a dislike of vegetables, often going back to childhood. Nevertheless, to lose weight effectively and improve our health, we need to face our demons and make eating some fruit and lots of vegetables the central part of every meal.

We know that our evolutionary history has designed us to function at our best on a 'predominantly plant-based diet' but what does this really mean? Should we just have an extra Brussels sprout at Christmas? Do we have to eat the token salad atop our take-away burger and fries? Sorry, not even close.

I used this phrase earlier in the book: "We are eating in a way that is completely out of kilter with our evolutionary design". Well, the simplest way to re-dress our out-of-kilter diet is to replace all the processed carbohydrate with fruit and lots of salad and vegetables. Real plant food is naturally low in calories but very high in nutrients, so by basing our diet around real plant foods we can start to lose weight effortlessly and begin to reverse the damage of a lifetime.

Why eat plants?

According to some of the world's leading scientists, low levels of fruit and vegetable consumption are intimately associated with rates of heart attacks, strokes and cancer (see page 242 for multiple references). In other words, the *more* fruit and vegetables we eat, the *less* chance we have statistically of developing any or all of these nasty conditions or diseases. A diet based on fruits and vegetables will help us lose weight and give us the best chance of improving our health over the long term.

Such remarkable health benefits are mainly down to the number and variety of phytochemicals contained in plants. These wonderful, naturally occurring chemicals are contained in fruits and salad/vegetables in large amounts and in enormous variety. Scientists are only just beginning to identify the chemical structure of some of these substances and are light years away from ever identifying the whole range of beneficial chemicals found in plants. Yet again, Nature has come up with the perfect solution to human health, if only we would take the time to see what is in front of our eyes. There are literally thousands of plants (and associated fruits) of all shapes, sizes and colours on this planet of ours, so it is high time we included just some of these wonder foods in our diet.

Eat fresh food in season if possible

Food is an expensive commodity but fruits and vegetables need not cost the Earth. Ideally, we should grow our own – a polytunnel at home or a local allotment is a great way to provide all the fruits and vegetables we need but, failing that, we should try to buy fruits and vegetables locally and in season. That means that in the UK, we should not be eating strawberries at Christmas or Brussels sprouts in July. In these enlightened times, we should support our local growers and farmers and enjoy their wonderful, fresh, seasonal produce throughout the year. Not only is this healthier and cheaper for us, it keeps our carbon footprint low and is good for the planet as well. I try to buy my veggies from nearby farmers' markets or my local supermarket, which has a very commendable policy of supporting local producers. Regardless of the source, we are blessed in this country with a huge variety of vegetables and fruits that are grown at different times of the year (Table 1).

Fruit

In his book 'Fit for Life', Sir Ranulph Fiennes states "Fruit is truly the panacea to good health". He's right, too, and fresh fruit will certainly form a very important part of our new, healthy diet in the future. However, certain fruits are very high in sugar, so it makes sense to be a little careful about how much fruit we eat in the early stages of our new, real food diet, particularly if we are diabetic or pre-diabetic. I recommend sticking at first to fruits that are not particularly sweet, such as the berries, e.g. raspberries, blueberries, strawberries, loganberries, blackberries, and tayberries. However, for most of us, the benefits of eating fruit will massively outweigh the risk that a small amount of natural fructose might have on our health.

So, which carbohydrates *should* we eat?

Many of us eat a diet that is packed full of carbohydrates. Many of our common foods such as breakfast cereals,

Table 1. A list of seasonal and vegetables available in the UK
(courtesy of www.lovebritishfood.co.uk)

	Spring	Summer	Autumn	Winter

Vegetables:	Asparagus
	Cauliflower
	Cucumber
	Jersey
	  Royal New
	  Potatoes
	Purple
	  Sprouting
	  Broccoli
	Radishes
	Savoy
	  Cabbage
	Sorrel
	Spinach
	Spring
	  Greens
	Spring
	  Onion
	Watercress
		Aubergine
		Beetroot
		Broad Beans
		Broccoli
		Carrots
		Courgettes
		Cucumber
		Fennel
		Fresh Peas
		Garlic
		Green Beans
		Lettuce and
		  Salad Leaves
		New potatoes
		Radishes
		Rocket
		Runner
		  Beans
		Salad Onions
		Sorrel
		Tomatoes
		Watercress
			Beetroot
			Carrot
			Celeriac
			Fennel
			Field
			  Mushrooms
			Kale
			Leeks
			Lettuce
			Marrow
			Potatoes
			Pumpkin
			Rocket
			Sorrel
			Squashes
			Sweetcorn
			Tomatoes
			Watercress
				Beetroot
				Brussels
				  Sprouts
				Cabbage
				Cauliflower
				Celeriac
				Chicory
				Fennel
				Jerusalem
				  Artichoke
				Kale
				Leeks
				Parsnips
				Potatoes
				Red
				  Cabbage
				Swede
				Turnips

Fruit:	Rhubarb	Blueberries
		Currants –
		  black, white
		  and red
		Elderflowers
		Greengages
		Loganberries
		Plums
		Raspberries
		Strawberries
		Tayberries
			Apples
			Blackberries
			Damsons
			Elderberries
			Pears
			Plums
			Quince
			Sloes
				Apples
				Pears

bread, soft drinks, beer, pastry, potatoes, rice, pasta, sweets, chocolates and cakes are packed full of carbohydrates. As carbohydrates are made from sugar, this means in effect that we are eating a diet that is almost exclusively sugar, which eventually ends up in our bloodstream as glucose or fructose.

However, this does not mean we should avoid all carbohydrates. Real, natural carbohydrate foods, such as certain fruits, salads, vegetables, a little brown rice, quinoa, seeds, nuts, even the odd baked potato for those who can cope with it, have none of the damaging effects of 'bad' carbs but instead should form the basis of a healthy, natural diet for the rest of our lives. We are designed to eat a predominantly vegetarian diet and provided such plant food is in its natural, unsullied state ("eat food from plants, not food made in a plant", as Michael Pollan says), the amount of carbohydrate is pretty much irrelevant. The most important aspect of dietary carbohydrate is the rate at which it ends up as glucose in the bloodstream. Real, natural plant foods have very little effect on our blood sugar levels, quite unlike most processed carbs, as we saw in the Glycaemic Index earlier in the chapter.

Choosing protein on the Back to Basics diet

Good quality proteins are a must on the Back to Basics diet. However, as we will be eating mostly plants, we won't need much in the way of extra protein, so can save money by eating this way as well. Here are some suggestions for sources of protein (recommended suppliers at the end of the book):

- *Meat and Poultry* – try to source local, organic chicken and meat and only eat meat in limited quantities (i.e. once or twice a week at most). As a happy by-product, this saves a lot of money, too.

- *Fish* – finding high-quality, ethically sourced fish can be a bit of a minefield but the situation is definitely improving, at least in the UK. Fish is a healthy and highly nutritious foodstuff and an excellent source of protein. Certain fish also provide high levels of very beneficial Omega 3 fatty acids.

- *Eggs* – a natural human food. Source high-quality, free-range organic eggs (or keep your own chickens) and enjoy a few times each week.

- *Dairy* – we are only designed to consume one type of dairy product, i.e. our mother's milk. We are not designed to consume the milk of other mammals and in particular, the milk from cows. Nevertheless, I do use a little skimmed milk in some of my fish recipes but I try to cut down on cow's milk products as much as possible. I do eat butter and cheese (feta in a Greek salad is a favourite) but rarely these days and only in very small quantities.

- *Legumes* – I love lentils and chickpeas but am not a huge fan of many other types of legume as they play havoc with my insides and I think there are generally better, more natural plant choices available. Nevertheless, I do eat legumes (see recipes) and with careful preparation, they are an excellent source of all the macronutrients and fibre we need in our diet. Vegans will certainly need to embrace legumes as a staple of their diet.

- *Nuts and Seeds* – I am not a fan of certain seeds (wheat, mostly) but flaxseed is an excellent vegetarian source of Omega 3, whilst nuts are a good source of healthy macronutrients and would have been a staple of our hunter-gatherer ancestors. For instance, walnuts are a good source of Omega 3 fatty acids and Brazil nuts contain selenium, one of our most important micronutrients, often lacking in the modern diet. Sunflower seeds and pumpkin seeds are delicious sprinkled over salads as well. Another seed I love is quinoa, which I eat two or three times a week.

Oils and Fats

We have discussed fats in some detail and have established that naturally occurring fats would have been an important part of our ancestral diet. However, the medical evidence suggests that an excessive amount of fat in the diet is not a great idea, so how should we approach eating fat on the Back to Basics diet?

Omega 6 : Omega 3 ratios

An easy way to achieve a correct Omega 6 : Omega 3 ratio

in our diet is to simply eat plenty of Omega 3 foods every day, e.g. walnuts, flaxseeds, oily fish. The Back to Basics diet is also an excellent foundation for the (rightly) popular Mediterranean diet and so I often make olive oil vinaigrette dressing for my salads. I am obsessed with the wonderful organic cold-pressed olive oils from the island of Crete, the best in the world as far as I am concerned. Nevertheless, I am aware that olive oil has a less than perfect Omega 6 : Omega 3 ratio (about 15:1, I think) and as in all oils, it is very energy rich, providing 9 calories of energy per gram of weight. So even though I love Cretan olive oil, I go easy on the quantity – just a teaspoon here and there.

Developing a healthy relationship with natural fat

In the Back to Basics diet, I have tried to strike a balance between eating less saturated fat (and a complete removal of trans fats) with an improved Omega 6 : Omega 3 ratio through a predominantly plant-based diet and *small* amounts of added virgin olive oil. In fact, we can gain virtually all our daily fat requirements from a small number of specific plant foods, such as flaxseed, walnuts, olives, avocados etc. Flaxseed, otherwise known as linseed, has been around for thousands of years but it is only recently that scientists have begun to realize just what a wonder food flax might be. It is naturally low in carbohydrate, bursting with wonderful phytonutrients and other good things but above all, it has high levels of Omega 3 fatty acids. It is now widely available in supermarkets and health food shops. A little organic virgin olive oil added to salads and vegetables completes the picture and removes any need for us to return to eating the trans fat-laden junk food of the past.

Overall, I believe this approach gives us the best chance of obtaining the essential nutrients from fat that we need whilst avoiding the dangers of a typical Western diet. This way, we can continue to lose weight and enjoy a new healthy relationship with 'good' fats at the same time.

Embracing real foods for easy weight loss

There are enough natural, healthy foods here to provide an endless variety of meals for the rest of our lives, so please don't worry that the Back to Basics diet is restrictive or difficult to follow. Similarly, try not to dwell on the foods missing from this list; leave those foods behind in the past, once and for all. Real food is delicious, cheap, healthy and the key to effortless lifelong weight loss. To make the switch to a plant-based, real food diet, we just need the courage to change; to change how we view food and to change how we buy and prepare food in the future. Most of all, we need to keep in mind how we are going to change, in body shape and in improved health, when we embrace these new wonderful foods.

5

There is more to this story than calories

*Our greatest glory is not in never falling, but in
getting up every time we do.*
Confucius

We have looked at the differences between real and processed
food and have established that the fundamental reason we
struggle with our weight is because our modern diet contains
more calories than we generally need. Unfortunately, we
evolved in a world where each and every calorie had to be
hunted or gathered, meaning our ancestors only survived
the lean times if they could store any excess calories as fat.
Today, this innate ability to store body fat has come back to
haunt us, especially in a world where highly calorific foods
are available to us 24/7.[1]

Although we each have our own unique genetic makeup
(so some of us put on weight more easily than others), the
ubiquitous availability of modern, processed foods makes it
very easy for us to eat too many calories and so gain weight.
Such foods not only contain high levels of calories but are
often tasty, relatively cheap and convenient as well, so we end
up eating lots of them! Even more disturbing is the power of

the marketing organization that keeps us buying these foods – that of the food industry. Suffice to say, if we live entirely on processed foods, it is fairly inevitable that our diet will contain an excess of calories.

However, the number of calories we consume each day is only part of the story. To get to the bottom of why we put on weight so easily we need to look beyond the simplistic 'calories in – calories out' model and the 'eat less, move more' mantra and delve a bit deeper into the workings of the human body. In doing so, we find it is the interplay of certain hormones that ultimately controls our appetite and how we manage the fat stores around our body.[2,3] Our modern diet upsets the workings of these hormones such that we develop various chronic conditions, including obesity.

Our body chemistry is identical to that of our Stone Age ancestors

In terms of how we digest and process our food, we are exactly the same as our earliest ancestors. Our body chemistry, identical to that of our hunter-gatherer predecessors, has evolved over eons of time under essentially the same diet, the diet everyone ate, for hundreds and thousands of years, before we ruined everything by inventing agriculture![4] The original human diet contained real, natural foods, low in calories but high in nutrients. For those just dipping into the book here for the first time, the typical ancestral diet comprised:

- High levels of naturally occurring plant material
- Reasonable amounts of animal protein and fat
- Very low levels of sugar (compared to our diet today)
- Absolutely no processed food!
- Relatively few calories (compared to our diet today)

This type of diet, when combined with plenty of daily exercise, kept our ancestors fit and healthy and gave them enough calories for their hard, demanding lives. During the summer months or after a successful hunt, they would have been able to lay down some fat reserves to see them through the hard times when food was scarce. However, as far as we can tell, they were not obese; they would have spent most of their lives perpetually hungry, frantically searching for their next meal.[5] To survive, they would have had to access and live off their fat reserves to keep them going until such time they could hunt or gather their next meal. So, part of our ancestral legacy is a fat double-edged sword – we are very efficient at storing fat (so we put on weight) but also have the means to use that fat for fuel (so we lose weight), when food is scarce. Today, most of us are experts at the former and not so adept at the latter.

Our body fat should act as a warehouse, not an archive

Our bodies still think we live in the Stone Age, so we lay down fat when food is plentiful, for use on a rainy day. When food is scarce, as it was throughout much of human history, we are supposed to live off this fat reserve until such time we can again find something to eat. Today, most of us never use our fat reserves – we just add to them all the time. However, if we can switch over to burning our body fat for a few hours each day (via an inherently low-calorie, low-processed-carb diet and periods of intermittent fasting), we can make use of our rainy day stores as Nature intended. We can then lose weight and avoid laying down excessive body fat in future. Much like taking stores out of a warehouse, we are supposed to access our body fat when food is scarce to tide us over until such time we are able to eat once more. Our body fat is not meant to be locked away forever in our tummy archive.

Our hormones hold the key to weight loss

Hormones control many of the biological processes we would probably rather forget – puberty, acne, menstruation, the menopause, obesity, sexual drive (or otherwise), growth, changes during pregnancy etc are all affected by hormones. Hormones are chemical messengers that are made in one part of the body but often tell a system somewhere else in the body to do something. By looking at how certain hormones work in and around the digestion of our food, we can begin to piece together the story of why we get so fat, so easily, on our modern diet.[6,7]

Our food hormones

There are a whole host of hormones that are intimately

involved in various aspects of obesity. Any number of these play an important role in the technical aspect of weight gain, e.g. *ghrelin*, a hormone secreted in the stomach that stimulates our appetite. In fact, one of the benefits of bariatric (weight loss) surgery seems to be the removal of ghrelin-producing cells when large chunks of the stomach are removed. Many other chemicals and hormones are also crucial in stimulating or blunting our appetites.

However, I want to concentrate on just two hormones because I believe they are the most important in the whole

HORMONES

- Hormones are proteins that are made in glands of the endocrine system, e.g. the pituitary, thyroid and adrenal glands, pancreas etc, before being secreted into the bloodstream to do their work somewhere else.
- Hormones control numerous processes in our bodies, e.g. puberty, acne, menstruation, the menopause.
- Hormones are directly involved in our obesity.
- The foods we eat in our modern diet (particularly processed carbohydrate) disturb certain hormones systems, e.g. insulin and leptin, resulting in weight gain.
- Although the calories in our diet ultimately decide whether or not we put on weight, if our 'food hormones' are disturbed by our modern diet it is very hard to avoid putting on weight (or subsequently to lose weight), however hard we try.

obesity story. One of these hormones is *insulin* which, in combination with excess calorie consumption, is a key factor in all aspects of obesity.[8,9] The other is called *leptin*, a hormone that controls appetite and hence one that often causes us to have 'eyes bigger than our stomachs'.

Leptin

The hormone leptin is secreted from our own fat cells and is supposed to tell us that our fat reserves are full, so stop eating.[10,11] Leptin levels are directly proportional to levels of adipose tissue, which in English means that the fatter the person, the more leptin they produce. In theory, *more* leptin should signal *less* eating but something has obviously gone wrong with our ability to respond to leptin, otherwise no one would be overweight or fat. From an evolutionary perspective, excess eating is costly and just plain unnecessary. In some ways, it would have been much easier for our earliest ancestors to survive the winter by becoming obese; they certainly wouldn't have starved to death with all that fat to live off. However, such obesity would have made it impossible for them to run away from predators or otherwise be a useful member of the tribe. So, evolution came up with leptin. Once sufficient fat reserves had been laid down, leptin would signal 'I'm full' and life would continue without having to eat all the time. Unfortunately, our modern diet plays havoc with our leptin response such that we don't respond to the signal to stop eating and hence tend to overeat instead.

Insulin

Insulin works in conjunction with another hormone to balance our blood sugar levels. Blood sugar? What has that got to do with putting on weight? Believe it or not, it is our blood sugar system, so badly messed up by our modern diet, that is key to understanding why so many of us have lost control of our weight.

Too many calories will certainly make us fat; however, insulin plays such a crucial role in determining our weight (and our health) that it is well worth spending some time now looking at this remarkable hormone in more detail.

Why blood sugar levels are so important

Many of our cells, tissues and organs are fussy about what they 'eat'. Our brains, in particular, rely almost exclusively on a regular supply of glucose in the blood, often just referred to as 'blood sugar'. There *is* an alternative energy source to glucose we could feed our brain known as a ketone body, a chemical manufactured in the liver from both dietary and stored body fats in times of starvation or if we eat a very low carbohydrate diet for a protracted period. (As an aside, a very low-carb diet, or 'ketogenic' diet, was originally designed to treat epilepsy but has become fashionable amongst the high-fat, low-carb diet set due to its perceived effect on reducing insulin levels). But we are designed to eat plants (which contain glucose), so under normal conditions we should feed our brains glucose, its preferred foodstuff, not ketones. However, we have to be careful about the source and quantity of that glucose; our brains are so fussy about the amount of glucose they need that blood sugar levels have to be maintained in an extremely narrow range of concentrations at all times or we are in trouble (Fig 5).

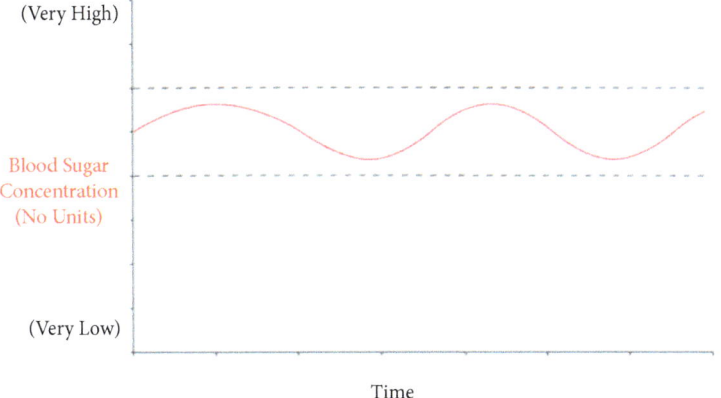

Fig 5. Blood sugar levels are maintained in a narrow range of concentrations at all times.

What concentration of blood sugar are we talking about? If we were to stir one teaspoon of table sugar into a 5-litre bucket of water (5 litres is roughly the total blood volume of an average person), we would approximate the ideal blood glucose concentration for our brain. Just a bit more sugar is toxic, whilst a slightly lower concentration also causes us problems, too. One teaspoon – that is not a lot of sugar.

A Back to Basics diet allows fine control of blood sugar

Imagine we are sitting down to a real food dinner, a meal consisting of the same types of food that fed our ancestors for hundreds and thousands of years. Eating this sort of food allows our hormones to balance our blood sugar levels easily and efficiently, just as Nature intended. By contrast, our modern high-sugar diet puts this blood sugar system under enormous pressure, which can lead directly to obesity.[12]

Our dinner complete, we settle onto the sofa to watch the latest box set. In between the belches and burps, the natural, real food from our meal is slowly digested. In particular, unprocessed plant food is difficult to break down, so the glucose from the plant food (plus the amino acids from proteins and fatty acids from fat) is slowly drip fed into the bloodstream in the hours following the meal. This is all perfectly natural and exactly how we are designed to process food.

Insulin gets to work

As the glucose passes into the bloodstream, our blood sugar concentration slowly starts to rise. We know this rise in blood sugar must be controlled or the brain will be damaged. Indeed, if our blood sugar levels get too high, a doctor will tell us we have *hyperglycaemia* (US: hyperglycemia) or too much sugar in the blood (Fig 6). Somehow, blood glucose levels have to be maintained at a sufficiently high concentration

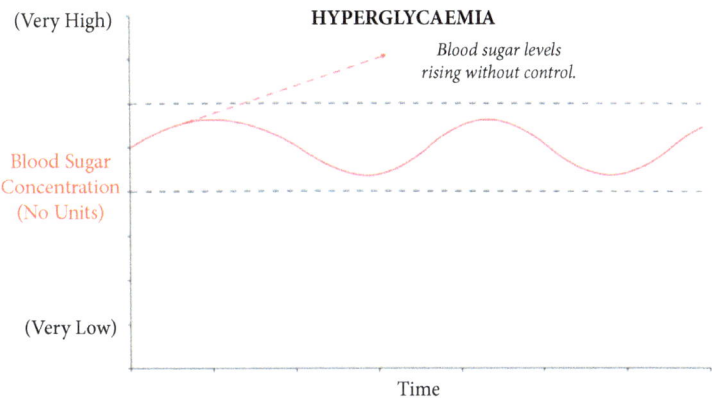

Fig 6. If blood sugar levels rise too much, we risk a dangerous condition known as 'hyperglycaemia'.

to satisfy the requirements of the brain and other cells and tissues, whilst at the same time kept within safe levels.

To get around this problem, the amazing power of evolution has come up with the hormone insulin to manage our blood sugar levels. Insulin stops blood sugar levels rising too much *by removing excess glucose* from the bloodstream.[13]

Our much abused pancreas

After a meal, biochemical sensing systems in the pancreas notice the rising levels of glucose in the blood. In response, cells in one part of the pancreas (beta cells) secrete insulin into the bloodstream. If the meal in question contained real, natural, unprocessed foods (mostly plants), only a small amount of insulin would be needed as such foods result in a relatively *slow rise in blood sugar levels*. And because we don't get a rapid spike in blood sugar concentration, the corresponding insulin response is minimal, too.

Once the insulin has done its work and blood sugar levels have dropped back to where they should be, insulin returns to a 'ticking over' background level in the bloodstream, ready to perform exactly the same role at the next meal (Fig 7):

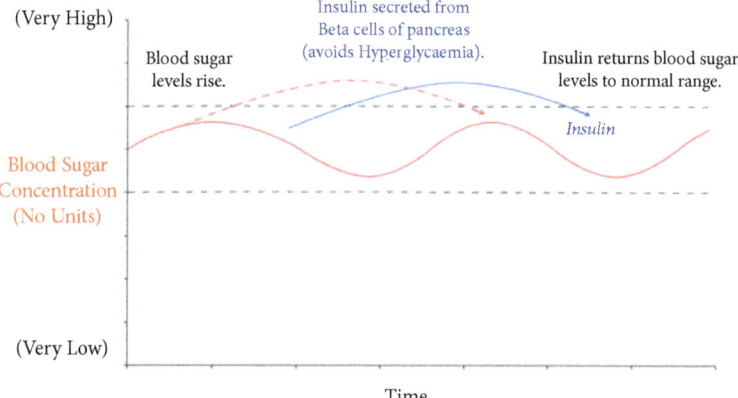

Fig 7. How insulin returns blood sugar levels to normal,
so avoiding hyperglycaemia

Too much insulin makes us fat

Insulin levels will rise when we eat all sorts of food but most insulin is secreted in response to eating sugar (e.g. processed carbohydrate). The more sugar we eat, the more insulin our pancreas has to produce. However, we know our blood sugar levels have to be kept at the equivalent of one teaspoon of sugar in our entire blood volume. So, where does this excess glucose go? Various cells and tissues will use some immediately but any remaining glucose will be stored in the body as a reserve of energy, available later when food is scarce. This is insulin's key role – excess blood glucose is swept out of the bloodstream and stored for a rainy day.[14]

So, the next question is, how and where is all this excess glucose stored? It is first stored in the liver and muscles in the form of *glycogen* (animal starch really), a polysaccharide of glucose and our main short-term energy source. However, once glycogen stores are full, any remaining glucose is stored as fat.

Insulin drives excess blood sugar to fat

Glycogen is evolution's answer to the sabre-toothed tiger; back in the Stone Age, when we needed to run away from something with big teeth fast, we used our glycogen reserve for immediate energy. These days, most of us can store about 400 grams of glycogen in total, which provides less than two hours worth of energy during strenuous exercise. If we run marathons twice a week or do a huge amount of heavy manual work, we will make use of our glycogen stores and so need to replenish them at every meal. Unfortunately, for most of us, our glycogen reserves are pretty much full all the time.

When glycogen stores are full, the body faces a quandary. Blood sugar levels still need to be controlled, so under the influence of insulin, any remaining glucose and triglycerides in the bloodstream are now stored as fat in various organs and in our fat cells (adipose tissue). The higher the levels of insulin, the more of this storage occurs. Yes, too much fat in our diet can make things worse (independent of insulin) but it is largely a myth that eating too much fat makes us fat. What *really* makes us overweight is the over-consumption of heavily processed, sugary foods throughout the day. Not only do we then eat too many calories but we also force insulin to work overtime by constantly having to sweep excess sugar from the bloodstream. This leads directly to weight gain because insulin stores excess sugar as fat.

To lose weight we need to keep our insulin levels low

Most of us eat in a way that keeps our insulin levels high, all day long. That is neither surprising nor our fault as we live in a world where food is everywhere we look, so we all tend to eat too much, too often. Nevertheless, we are perfectly adapted to survive periods of famine by living off the fat reserves around our body. Unfortunately, we are not very adept at this side of our fat metabolism these days. However, if we look deeper into the action of insulin, we find the secret 'switch' that allows us to start burning body fat, so that we can lose weight once and for all.

Imagine it is several hours since our last meal – our stomachs are now empty and we are starting to get hungry. Insulin levels are low because we are not consuming food – there is no need for high levels of insulin in the bloodstream at this point. When insulin levels are low, the biochemical process that accesses our fat reserves is switched 'on'. This fat burning process is called lipolysis, evolution's answer to living in a world where food supply was decidedly intermittent.

When insulin levels are low, we are able to break down our body fat to power our lives until our next meal, whenever that might be, exactly as we are designed to work.

However, when insulin levels are high (as is the case for most of us all day long) lipolysis is switched 'off', meaning our bodies are unable to burn fat.[15,16] Therefore, if we spend our lives permanently 'insulinated', i.e. with high levels of insulin in our bloodstream, it is hard to lose weight, regardless of calorie consumption. To burn fat away from around our bodies and re-gain control of our own health destiny, we need to keep our insulin levels low as much as possible.

What happens if we don't eat for a while?

Our ancestors did not starve to death in the lean times, even if they couldn't find anything to eat for a day or two. They would have been very hungry but they survived because they were able to live off their fat reserves, just as evolution intended. This is one of many reasons why humans are the most successful species on the planet.

However, what happens to blood sugar levels if we don't eat for a while? In theory they could fall too low but evolution has an answer for this as well. When blood sugar levels start to drop, another hormone (called glucagon) is secreted from a different part of the pancreas; glucagon releases glucose from storage (from glycogen in the liver, mostly) to re-balance the concentration of glucose in the blood to the correct level. In fact, glucagon can keep our blood sugar topped up for about three days before we need to eat again. Glucose can even be made from other bits and pieces of protein digestion if need be as well. Suffice to say, we are perfectly capable of keeping our blood sugar from falling too low (a condition known as hypoglycaemia) by using our own biochemistry.

Insulin and glucagon control our blood sugar levels

So between them, insulin and glucagon work in harmony to control our blood sugar levels (Fig 8).

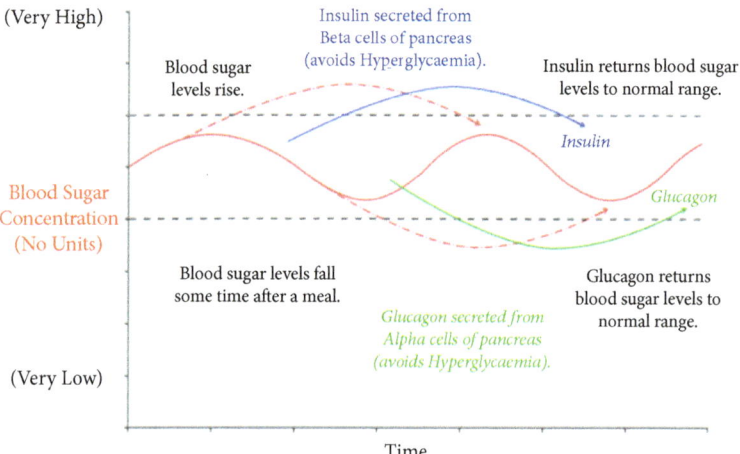

Fig 8. Insulin and glucagon combine in a feedback system to control blood sugar concentration at all times.

Insulin and glucagon are designed to work as a fine tuning mechanism, ticking away in the background, balancing our blood sugar levels here and there after infrequent, low-sugar meals. The key point is this – under normal circumstances, we are extremely *sensitive* to these two hormonal signals. Together, insulin and glucagon are more than capable of keeping our blood sugar at the correct level.[17]

We don't need to eat all the time

Unfortunately, our modern diet asks insulin to function much like the inexperienced Captain of an extremely large boat. The Captain turns the boat to starboard but realizes that he has overdone it because the boat turns far more than he wanted. He spins the wheel the other way, only to find he has over-corrected again, leading to the ship swinging wildly to and fro, either side of the intended course. This is what happens to our insulin system when we eat frequent, high-sugar meals; the rush of insulin can often remove *too much* glucose, resulting in a rather dramatic swing in blood sugar back down towards hypoglycaemia. We recognize the symptoms as suddenly feeling woozy and unwell, so we rush off for another high sugar snack a few hours later. Insulin levels shoot back up, excess glucose is again swept out of the bloodstream and we are once more pushed towards hypoglycaemia. Eating high–sugar meals inevitably leads to this wild swing in blood glucose levels (see Fig 9).

By contrast, a real food, plant-based diet with plenty of time between meals allows insulin to remain at a background level for most of the day, only being secreted from the pancreas in very small quantities during and shortly after our (infrequent) meals of unprocessed food. We are meant to be in a state of low insulin for most of the time.

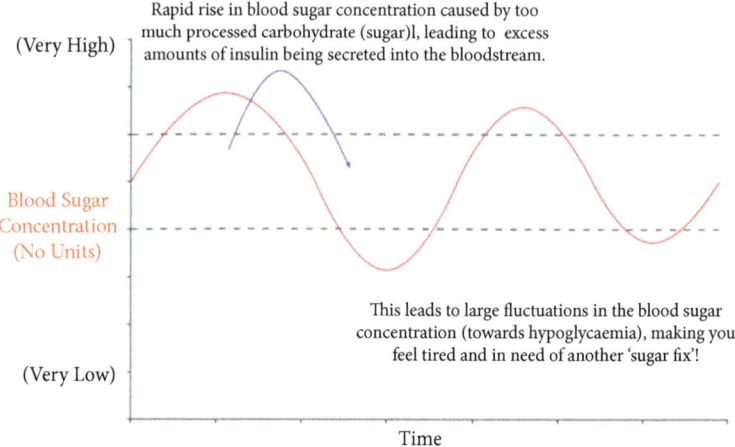

*Fig 9. Fluctuations in blood sugar concentration caused by excess
processed carbohydrate (and other rich foods!)*

The Back to Basics diet and insulin

Myriad fad and extreme diets exist these days but the most
effective way to lose weight and boost health is to combine a
real food, plant-based diet (which naturally reduces calorie
consumption and provides lots of health-giving nutrients)
with a reduction in the *number* of meals we eat, such that
insulin levels are kept low as much as possible. If we can cut
down the number of meals we eat to, say, two a day, and add
in daily activity, we really put the mockers on insulin and
give ourselves the best chance of changing the bad habits of
a lifetime.

The Back to Basics programme combines delicious,
healthy, natural real foods with daily activity and a little

intermittent fasting to control insulin levels. Most of the day will be spent in a state of low insulin, when lipolysis is activated and we burn fat, rather than in high insulin, where we constantly try to put on weight instead. Everything calms down and by managing our diet and lifestyle in this way, we put the final nail in the coffin of our obesity, once and for all.

Insulin resistance

Rather than being sensitive to insulin, many of us who are overweight have become *resistant* to the message insulin is trying to send.[18,19,20] Such *insulin resistance* is a key element in both weight gain and Type 2 diabetes and also underpins the difficulties we encounter when we try to lose weight. What causes insulin resistance is still a topic of debate. The latest research seems to point to the culprit being ever increasing levels of fat in and around our organs, which interfere with the normal action of insulin.[21,22] Other theories suggest that something in our modern diet is upsetting the normal mechanism of insulin, so that far too much insulin is produced, far too often, leading again to insulin resistance.[23] Either way, the important point is that we are no longer responding to insulin the way we should. The concept of insulin resistance is pretty much central to any theory about why our modern diet makes us fat, so let's look at this crucial aspect of our body chemistry in a bit more detail.

MANAGING OUR INSULIN

- Imagine an old-fashioned signal box on the side of a railway line, full of those huge levers that switch the points. A rather Victorian gentleman, complete with waistcoat, peaked cap and bushy moustache, is grasping one of those levers on our behalf.

- We have just woken up – glucagon levels are *high*, insulin levels are *low* (we don't need insulin when we are asleep – there isn't any excess glucose over night because we are fasting). We are now primed for weight loss. If we don't eat anything for a few hours, our energy needs have to be met from our fat and glycogen stores, mediated by low insulin levels, rather than from food.

- Imagine instead that we have just tumbled out of bed, put on the kettle and grabbed a bowl of cereal and a couple of rounds of white toast, with butter and marmalade. What happens in the signal box now? The signalman will switch over our body chemistry from a *fasting* state (with glucagon in the ascendancy) to a *fed* state (where *insulin* is secreted in response to food, especially if we eat a high carbohydrate meal).

- In the fed state, our body wants to *store* food energy. Consequently, it is very *hard to lose weight*. We have to wait for a few hours after a meal for insulin to return to a background level before lipolysis kicks in and we can live off our warehouse of fat once again.

Insulin resistance – it's all to do with our genes

We are able to control our blood sugar levels through the subtle action of insulin and glucagon after infrequent meals of real food. By design, blood sugar levels are supposed to be fairly stable. However, on our modern, high-sugar diet, we hammer our blood sugar levels all day long, so all our poor old pancreas can do in response is unleash a tsunami of insulin in an attempt to stave off imminent hyperglycaemia. This unnaturally high level of insulin not only means we are constantly trying to store our food energy as fat but also affects our ability to sense insulin in the first place.

Our genes control everything and tell our bodies when to 'make something'. This includes making insulin receptors, clever cellular structures that recognize insulin and allow the insulin molecule to dock to the cell surface of the various liver, muscle and adipose (fat) cells. However, if we bombard these receptors all day long with too much insulin, the genes that control their production get turned off, simply because they are trying to protect the cells from this unnaturally high level of insulin. We can soak up quite a lot of excess insulin by exercising, probably because exercise uses glycogen, which can then be topped up via the action of insulin without problem. However, if we are sedentary, the insulin in our bloodstream eventually causes our insulin receptor genes to shut down, leading directly to insulin resistance.[14]

Now we have a problem. At this point, more and more insulin has to be produced to achieve the same reduction in blood sugar concentration that we used to achieve with a much lower concentration of insulin when we were insulin sensitive. This overload of insulin eventually leads to *hyperinsulinaemia*, which can lead to some or all of the medical conditions listed here:

- High blood pressure (hypertension)
- Inhibition of lipolysis (fat burning)
- Inflammation, leading to higher risk of cardiovascular disease, strokes, cancers etc
- Impaired glucose tolerance (makes sense – too much glucose in the blood)
- Worn out pancreatic beta cells
- Increased hunger, so we eat too much (via hypoglycaemia)
- Pre-disposition to Type 2 diabetes

Insulin resistance and obesity

When I started the research for this book, I soon discovered the theory that obesity is caused by excess carbohydrate consumption, leading to elevated insulin levels, leading in turn to hyperinsulinaemia, then insulin resistance and the subsequent storage of fat. This is all explained in the book 'Good Calories, Bad Calories' by Gary Taubes (see bibliography). This is a controversial theory, which is still regarded as a bit left field, but it goes something like this:

Excess carbs → excess insulin → hyperinsulinaemia
→ *insulin resistance* → obesity

There are two sides to a coin, of course, so the more mainstream argument is this:

Too many calories → obesity → *insulin resistance* → hyperinsulinaemia

The key point here is *insulin resistance*; whichever way you spin it, it is insulin resistance, in combination with a high-calorie diet, which underpins the current obesity epidemic and the concurrent epidemic of Type 2 diabetes. However, such academic musings can be left to the professionals because all that concerns us is what to eat each day. It is our highly processed, high-sugar diet that makes us fat; not only do we eat too many calories, we also send our highly sensitive blood sugar control mechanism haywire, leading eventually to obesity and insulin resistance. This is why tackling insulin resistance is such a key part of the Back to Basics diet.

Type 2 diabetes

If our insulin resistance gets to the stage where we can no longer produce enough insulin to keep control of our own blood sugar, a doctor will tell us that we have Type 2 diabetes (T2D). Our pancreas will probably be worn out as well, from making all the extra insulin. Our own insulin has done its best but we can no longer keep a lid on the sugar levels in our bloodstream without extra help from the doctor. So, if you have or think you have T2D, please go and see your doctor for a check-up. I am not a medical doctor, so the treatment of T2D is outside the scope of this book. To get a doctor's view on how to reverse diabetes, I thoroughly recommend the excellent book *Reverse your Diabetes* by Dr David Cavan, one of the UK's leading specialists in diabetes treatment. Those with T2D need to work closely with their doctor when beginning this or any other diet as diabetic medication can cause hypoglycaemia if sugar is suddenly stripped out of the diet. Nevertheless, it is now clear that weight loss is the key to reversing T2D. Not everyone will be able to alter the status of their diabetes without continued medication but there is good evidence that significant weight loss (through this or any other sensible diet) can make it entirely possible to regain control of blood sugar levels and put T2D into remission.

The latest thinking on the causes of Type 2 diabetes

Thanks to the work of Professor Roy Taylor's team at Newcastle, the evidence now seems unequivocal that T2D is ultimately caused by a build-up of visceral fat in and around the liver and the pancreas.[24] It seems such fat interferes with the action of insulin, resulting in insulin resistance and a failure to control our own blood sugar.

We all have our own unique visceral fat 'tipping point'; in other words, we each have a genetically pre-determined level of visceral fat beyond which we develop T2D. Some of us can tolerate more visceral fat than others; however, if we keep on gaining weight we are all at risk of developing T2D. I should stress that there is mounting evidence that a sensible diet and exercise programme can *most definitely* reverse this situation, such that T2D can be put into remission.[25]

Regaining insulin sensitivity on the Back to Basics programme

The Back to Basics programme is designed to achieve two key changes; firstly, by re-establishing a healthy relationship with real food, we naturally reduce our calorie intake and so get our energy intake in balance once more. Secondly, the choice of foods, meal plans and, particularly, the timing of the meals helps us regain sensitivity to insulin. As our insulin sensitivity improves, we will need less insulin than we needed before and so can keep our insulin levels low as well. Not only will our calorie intake be under control but we will make much better use of our stored fat (via low insulin levels) and so will lose excess body fat, rather than adding to it all the time.

The Back to Basics Diet allows the insulin/glucagon system to work correctly. By changing what we eat, together with making subtle changes to when we eat, we can regain control of our blood sugar levels and avoid the wild swings in blood sugar concentration characteristic of our modern, high-sugar diet.

Stay young forever – another reason to control insulin?

Exciting new science coming out of America might make a 'low-insulin' lifestyle even more enticing.

Ageing has always been thought of as a natural part of life. However, an eminent American scientist (Professor Cynthia Kenyon) has recently identified two genes in a worm (!) that might hold the key to a dramatically longer life for all of us, free from disease and all the normal signs of ageing, including getting fat.[26,27]

Genes are sections of our DNA that contain a code, which when turned on tell our body to 'do something' or 'make something'. Remarkably, it seems that if we change what we eat (yes, back to real food and away from insulin-spiking processed carbs and sugar), we might be able to control these particular genes so that we can delay ageing and avoid many of the normal symptoms of old age. OK, these genes were found in worms but it seems likely they exist in humans as well.

Professor Kenyon named the first of the two genes the 'Grim Reaper' because it seemed to code for all the normal signs of ageing. However, the second gene, nicknamed 'Sweet Sixteen', had an amazing ability to confer youth in its host. It seems that an active Grim Reaper gene stops the youthful Sweet Sixteen gene from working, so ageing happens as per normal. Here is the startling fact, though – the Grim Reaper gene codes for a protein that allows certain cells and tissues to recognize a particular hormone, one with an identical molecular shape to insulin![28]

Although there is a long way to go with the science yet, it seems highly likely these two genes do exist in humans. So, if we can somehow switch off, or at least restrict, the action of the Grim Reaper gene by making *less insulin*, the Sweet

Sixteen gene can start to work. This will lead to a remarkable cascade of good chemical reactions throughout the body, which to all intents and purposes keeps us young. However, if we eat in a way that keeps the Grim Reaper gene switched 'on', the Sweet Sixteen gene will be turned off. We will then age and get fat as per normal, and risk all those nasty diseases we have already discussed. So, by eating so that we minimize our insulin response, we might be able to stave off old age, at least for a while. One day, no doubt, we'll be able to take a pill, which will let us live to 100 with the body of a 30-year-old; in the meantime, this seems like another very good reason to adopt a low-insulin lifestyle.

6

Changing when we eat – the final piece in the weight loss jigsaw

Mastering others is strength. Mastering yourself is true power.
Lao Tzu

Changing *when* we eat is the final step in unlocking the secret of permanent weight loss, which is why I am about to suggest a radically different approach to meal times. Changing when we eat is just a polite way of saying we should eat less often. The good news is that eating less often does *not* mean we are going to starve ourselves; a real food, plant-based diet ensures we remain full all day long, even if we eat fewer meals than we used to do in the past. Reducing the number of meals we eat is not a new idea, as 'fasting' has been practised around the world for thousands of years. Nevertheless, there has been a surge of interest recently in how eating less often might aid weight loss, resulting in the popular dietary protocol known as 'intermittent fasting'. I am a huge fan of intermittent fasting as by altering the number, content and timing of our meals we can use our body chemistry to best advantage, rather than remaining over-caloried and insulinated by eating all the time.

Eat six meals a day? Not if we want to lose weight

Our modern diet makes us fat because it contains too many calories and because it causes our insulin levels to rise too much, too often. This is particularly true if our meals contain mostly processed carbohydrates and sugar. Excess calories are a problem but too much insulin in the bloodstream contributes to obesity and eventually makes us insulin resistant, which can lead to lots of unwanted medical issues.

Nevertheless, one of the most depressing pieces of advice I see in the diet literature is the recommendation to eat five or six small meals every couple of hours throughout the day.[1] This, we are told, is necessary 'to keep our metabolism up' so we can 'stabilize our blood sugar levels'. Well, I appreciate the sentiment but unfortunately, this advice is fundamentally wrong. Eating every couple of hours is certainly not how you or I are designed to eat.[2]

Keeping our metabolism up?

We had a brief look at metabolism earlier in the book, where we saw how it is generally divided into two main categories, i.e. catabolism and anabolism.[3] If you remember, catabolism is the breakdown and digestion of food to constituent parts, e.g. carbohydrate to glucose, fats to free fatty acids and glycerol and proteins to amino acids. In turn, anabolism is the process whereby these constituent parts are used to build up new cellular components, using the energy released during catabolism.

So, which metabolism are we going to keep up if we eat every couple of hours? The answer is catabolism, followed by anabolism. Uh oh, alarm bells. What is the main hormone involved in anabolism? Insulin! So, by eating all the time (eating six meals a day is definitely eating all the time), we just risk eating too many calories and making ourselves permanently insulinated, both of which do tremendous damage to our waistlines and our health.

What about stabilizing blood sugar levels?

We know the human brain requires a constant blood glucose concentration roughly equivalent to one teaspoon of sugar in total blood volume. Do we need to eat constantly to maintain this blood sugar level? No, we are more than capable of maintaining that blood sugar concentration ourselves via our biochemistry (and without the dubious benefit of constant eating), just as evolution worked out long ago. Although diabetics may have need for more frequent meals, it is a myth that the rest of us have to eat all the time to manage our blood sugar levels. We are designed, by evolution, to function at our best on a lifestyle of daily activity and infrequent meals.[4] It would certainly help us to lose weight if these meals were eaten at the same time each day but constant eating is simply not necessary to control blood sugar levels. To help explain all this, we need to return to our old friends insulin and glucagon to see how these remarkable hormones work together to balance our blood sugar without us having to eat all the time.

Our liver holds the key

Imagine we have just woken up and got out of bed, ready for the new day. We know that insulin and glucagon are closely tied and when one hormone is elevated, the other drops to a background level. We haven't eaten for several hours, so during the night our insulin levels have gone down and therefore our glucagon levels have gone up:

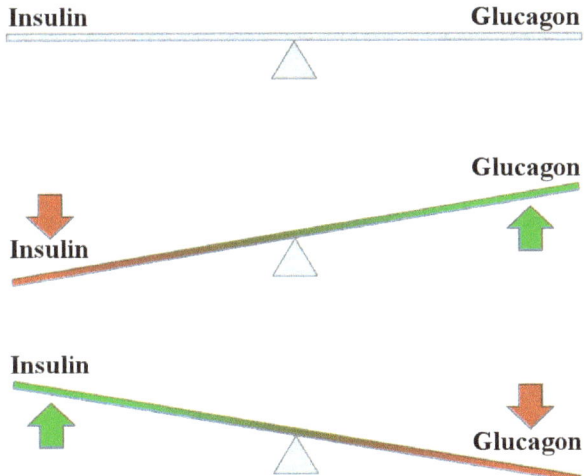

We saw earlier that glucagon was able to keep blood sugar levels stable by effecting the breakdown of glycogen to glucose and the production of 'new' glucose from other bits and pieces of digestive by-product. As glucagon levels climb during the night, two complementary processes take place in the liver, both of which produce glucose to top up our blood sugar to the correct level.[5] The first of these processes involves stored glycogen being broken down to glucose; the second process, with the wonderful name of *gluconeogenesis*, is when new glucose is made from other non-carbohydrate bits, such as amino acids, glycerol, lactate etc. So, when our blood sugar starts to drop during the night, the liver balances the breakdown of glycogen with the production of glucose to keep our blood sugar level at the right concentration. It is a bit like the central heating thermostat in our house – we set a temperature we wish to be maintained (i.e. our blood sugar level) and the system turns the heating on and off as necessary to maintain that temperature. So, a low insulin/high glucagon ratio not only enables us to burn the fat from around our bodies so we lose weight, it keeps our blood sugar levels stable as well.

So, how do six small meals a day smooth out blood sugar? They don't do anything of the sort, of course. Eating that often forces us to burn glucose rather than body fat and risks us eating too many calories, too. We will probably spend the whole day permanently insulinated as well.

Changing when we eat to maximize low insulin levels

High levels of insulin in the bloodstream block access to the vast number of calories we have locked away in our fat by inhibiting lipolysis, so making weight loss very difficult.[6] Even worse, elevated insulin levels make us add to our already bulging fat reserves and can make us ill through inflammation, insulin resistance and Type 2 diabetes. We might even shorten our lives by switching on the Grim Reaper gene as well. So, it just seems common sense to minimize the time we spend insulinated as much as possible. However, a low level of insulin (or if you like, a correspondingly high level of glucagon) allows us to manage our blood sugar levels quite happily, whilst allowing us to burn body fat (so we lose weight) at the same time.[7,8]

It would help if we could minimize our insulin response through our diet; we can certainly help things along by moving away from processed foods and returning to a plant-based, low processed food diet. However, to get our insulin levels really under control, we need to go further and employ a little fasting as well. This way, we can spend far more hours in the day in low insulin (when fat burning is optimized) rather than in a state of high insulin when our ability to lose weight is severely impaired. In so doing, we fit the final piece into the weight loss jigsaw and markedly improve our chances of life long, permanent weight loss. By tipping the odds in our favour this way, we will finally stop swimming against the tide of our own body chemistry.

The Back to Basics programme helps change when we eat

We don't need to go back in time to the Stone Age to eat correctly or return to a healthy weight. By switching to a plant-based, real food diet and making some subtle changes to our mealtimes, we can easily control our calorie intake, get all the nutrients we need and keep our insulin levels at a low, background level for most of the day. The Back to Basics programme is designed to help with all these factors in a simple and straightforward manner, so we can forget about the nuts and bolts of the science and instead get on with losing weight and enjoying life as much as possible.

How can we change when we eat in order to help us lose weight? Well, to get the ball rolling, imagine for a moment that we are looking at the clock face of a 24-hour clock (Fig 10):

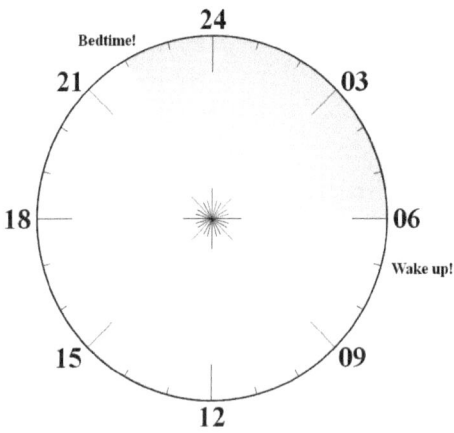

Fig 10. A 24-hour clock face

Let's imagine we have just woken up at 7.00 am after a good night's sleep. Our last meal was dinner at 7.00 pm the night before, so our blood insulin levels are now low (we have effectively been fasting for twelve hours). As insulin levels fall, glucagon levels rise, so our blood sugar levels have been topped up through the night as discussed earlier. What happens now if we wander into the kitchen in our dressing gown and grab a bowl of cornflakes and some white toast with butter and marmalade?

Everything changes. First of all, we unleash a tsunami of insulin from the pancreas in an attempt to remove all the excess sugar we have just dumped into our bloodstream from our sugary breakfast. We also risk sending our blood sugar levels yo-yoing up and down because such large amounts of insulin can sweep out too much glucose in one go, dropping us temporarily into hypoglycaemia. This makes us feel light-headed and a bit unwell, so we crave some more sugary food so we can 'balance our blood sugar' and off we go again. And it is very, very hard to lose weight when we are insulinated, as we now know.

Using daily activity to our best advantage

Instead of eating a big sugary breakfast first thing in the morning, how about we give breakfast a miss for a couple of hours and go out for a jog instead? Or cycle to work? Or walk the kids to school? Let's have a look at what happens when we delay eating our first meal of the day for a few hours.

We know that when we wake up in the morning, insulin levels are low and glucagon levels are high. But today we have resisted the urge to eat a large breakfast and have instead pulled on our trainers and gone out of the front door. It's our choice but we will either end up at work (if we walk or cycle to work) or back at the front door having walked the kids to school or otherwise exercised out in the fresh air for maybe 45 minutes to an hour. This isn't a problem because today we got out of bed an hour earlier than usual, so we could get our morning activity fix.

Where is the energy coming from for this early morning activity? We haven't eaten breakfast yet so we need to dip into our reserves instead, i.e. glycogen and fat. This is all accessed quite naturally through our low-insulin/high-glucagon state, exactly how evolution has designed our bodies to work. By allowing our insulin levels to remain low at the beginning of the day, we are able to use our reserves to provide loads of energy for even extended periods of activity. Meanwhile, our blood sugar levels are taken care of by the breakdown of glycogen and if necessary, a smidgen of gluconeogenesis, all controlled by the interplay of insulin and glucagon. Having returned from our morning excursion, we shower, get on our bike and cycle gently to work, burning a few more calories in the process. We are now free to enjoy a healthy breakfast or brunch at some point later in the morning.

Living life in low insulin

By taking most of our daily activity in the morning and not eating beforehand, we have worked with our body chemistry to access the stored energy from around our body, just as Nature intended. This early morning period is the ideal time to get active and also the time when we should not be eating. It is the time of day when we have naturally low insulin/high glucagon levels and so are primed to burn fat, not store fat.

What happens when we eventually have something

to eat? We now switch over to what the scientists call the 'fed' state and insulin once again regains the upper hand for a while. However, this is quite normal.[9] If we stick to foods such as vegetables, berry fruits, lean meat/poultry, fish, eggs and healthy, natural fats in small quantities, we will not generate an excessive insulin response. Instead, we will only require a small amount of insulin to smooth out our blood sugar levels – a few hours later, insulin will again take a back seat and glucagon levels will start to rise once more. This is what happened every day for millions of years whenever our ancestors ate something, before we messed it all up by over-processing food and eating sugar.

Using changes in mealtimes to really get rid of the flab

The more activity we can take each day, the easier it will be for us to get our calorie intake in balance without having to eat small portions of food.[10] If we can manage our insulin levels as well, we are doing exactly what we need to do to ensure we lose weight effectively. Having eaten a late (ish) breakfast or an early lunch, our insulin levels should have returned to a low background level by the afternoon.

Can we now fit in some more activity? Yes, because it is now time for our cycle ride home from work or our walk to collect the kids from school or our afternoon session at the gym. Once again, we are using our body chemistry to our advantage and are no longer swimming against the tide of insulin. By using our low insulin phases of the day in this way, we are working with our body chemistry, rather than eating all the time and hence trying to lose weight in a permanent state of elevated blood insulin.

How many meals should we eat?

Most of us have grown up eating three meals a day plus the odd snack and would regard this as a perfectly normal way to eat. Some of us (hand up here) might also add a few pints after work and a takeout on the way home to the list of 'normal' eating too. However, we know that over-eating is unnecessary and potentially damaging to our health, so how often should we really eat? Well, as always in matters of human nutrition, there is no absolute answer. Nevertheless, I want to suggest a different way to structure eating through the day by first giving breakfast a miss. Too many of us start the day by getting out of bed and immediately reaching for sugar in the form of breakfast cereal, white bread, pastries, sugary tea, marmalade etc. This dumps a huge amount of sugar and calories into the bloodstream first thing in the morning and causes a massive spike in blood insulin levels, even before we have got dressed.

If we resist the urge to eat straightaway and instead get active (by cycling or walking to work, for instance), we can extend our overnight fast and so keep insulin levels low for a few more hours of the day. Once we have got to work (or back at home after our morning activity), we can reward ourselves with a healthy, tasty breakfast or brunch later in the morning. This meal can effectively replace both breakfast and lunch and can be quite hearty, provided it consists of plentiful real foods (there are some suggestions for brunches and portable meals to take to work later in the book). We can then get on with our day, safe in the knowledge that we have taken a huge step towards a much healthier, slimmer way of life. In the afternoon, we can enjoy a healthy snack of fresh fruit or raw vegetables before looking forward to a delicious supper of healthy, tasty real foods and perhaps a glass of wine. This is after we have cycled home from work, of course ☺.

I will cover all this in more detail in Part 2 but I suggest we just try to eat two meals a day (plus one mid-afternoon snack). Ideally, the first meal should be taken late in the morning or at lunchtime, after we have done some sort of morning activity – walking is fine. Our second meal should be taken in the early evening, again after some more exercise. I recommend a snack of fruit, veggies etc at some point in the afternoon. At first sight this may sound restrictive but it really isn't and there is a virtually unlimited range of meals that can be put together around this template. Similarly, there is no need to eat small portions, the downfall of virtually every type of traditional diet. All we are trying to do is maximize the time we are best able to burn our own fat, whilst making sure that when we *do* eat, we eat plenty of highly nutritious, naturally low-calorie foods. This way, we will give ourselves the best possible chance of losing weight and keeping that weight off long-term. Here is a suggested timetable for a typical day on the Back to Basics diet:

Alarm goes off	Time to get up!
Early morning	*ACTIVITY* – Walk to work, cycle to work, walk the kids to school, walk around the park etc
Late morning – lunchtime	*EAT* – Time for the first meal of the day (one meal of healthy, nutritious, predominantly plant-based food). Take a packed 'brunch' to work
Mid-afternoon	*SNACK* – Fruit, veggies, some hummus perhaps?
Late afternoon	*ACTIVITY* – Walk home from work, cycle home from work, walk the kids back from school, walk around the park etc
Early evening	*EAT* – Time for dinner. Eat at the table, enjoy a glass of wine etc

Eating to suit our own lifestyle

We all need to work our mealtimes around our particular lifestyle, as the time of day we eat is less important than the number and content of meals we eat in total, provided we try to eat at roughly the same time each day. For instance, if we were to get up at dawn and then do two or three hours of hard labour (a farmer, for instance), we might eat our breakfast before 9.00 a.m. On another day, we might have a lie-in, then get up and go for a walk or go to the gym or go for a bike ride and so not eat much before normal lunchtime.

In both cases, we are playing by the rules because activity comes before eating. This just keeps us in our overnight low-insulin phase as long as possible before we 'break our fast'; in so doing, we give ourselves the best chance of burning fat before we start to consume calories once again. We will cover this in more detail in Part 2.

New thinking on intermittent fasting

What I am proposing here is my interpretation of intermittent fasting. Fasting works on many levels but in terms of weight loss, fasting is very simply the best way to achieve low insulin levels, with all the ensuing benefits to our health that we have already discussed. There has been a surge of interest in fasting recently, as it might possibly be the most effective technique there is for successful weight loss and improved health. There are many ways to fast, ranging from daily fasts (as recommended here) to two-day fasts and water-only fasts, right through to multi-day fasts lasting many weeks. Many of the more extreme fasts require medical supervision but under these circumstances, such extended fasts seem to be extraordinarily effective in reducing obesity and even reversing Type 2 diabetes. Much of the new thinking on intermittent fasting has been driven by a Canadian doctor called Dr Jason Fung, a nephrologist (kidney specialist) and an expert in the treatment of obesity and Type 2 diabetes through fasting and associated dietary protocols. His writing on this subject is both very good and very popular and I highly recommend his work to those interested in learning more about the ancient art of fasting for health.[11,12] Fasting works on many different levels; in terms of weight loss, fasting obviously restricts our calorie intake but also allows insulin levels to drop substantially, thereby enabling us to access our fat reserves via lipolysis. Regular fasting not only keeps insulin levels under control but also encourages insulin sensitivity, one of the main aims of the Back to Basics diet. Fasting has been shown time and again to be highly effective in achieving improved health and permanent weight loss.[13–17]

Many diets employ intermittent fasting in some form or another but here I recommend daily fasting in conjunction with a Back to Basics, real food diet. I recommend a cautious approach to fasting, so I suggest just giving breakfast a miss and only eating in a smaller segment of the day. This is the most sensible approach in the first instance and although there are numerous other fasting techniques out there, fasting for a few hours each day should be the first port of call for those following the Back to Basics diet. Feel free to experiment with other forms of fasting if you wish but the limited daily fasting I recommend here is based on sound biochemical principles and really helps us to lose weight.

By squeezing our eating into a smaller period of the day, we avoid switching our insulin system 'on' first thing in the morning with a sugary breakfast and then keeping it high all day long by grazing on processed food and junk food. With a bit of practice, we can soon forget about our sugary breakfast and instead replace it with some morning activity. We can then eat a healthy, nutritious, low-calorie breakfast a bit later. With a bit more practice, we can delay this late breakfast by an hour or two and turn it into a brunch instead. This way, we can really start to maximize our ability to lose weight. By condensing all our eating into a small period of the day, we spend just a few hours gently insulinated but far longer in a state of low insulin, where we can burn fat, lose weight and take huge steps towards a much healthier lifestyle. By following a daily fast in combination with a plant-based, real food diet, we can return to a way of life that evolution has spent millions of years perfecting; instead of constantly gaining weight and damaging our health via a diet of processed foods, we can become slim, fit and a lot happier, too.

7

New ideas and ancient knowledge

Success is not final, failure is not fatal:
it is the courage to continue that counts.
Winston Churchill

We have now seen how our modern diet is completely out of kilter with our body chemistry. There are numerous reasons for this, some of which we discussed earlier; nevertheless, many of the factors that lead to obesity are now conveniently grouped together under the heading of something called the 'obesogenic environment'. This rather clumsy phrase just means our genes still think we live in the Stone Age (where we are expected to eat a low calorie, intermittent diet) but our modern environment, with its fast food outlets and convenience foods 24/7, tends to encourage excess calorie consumption and inactivity. The result is a complex web of diet and lifestyle issues that, despite our best intentions, often lead to us putting on weight. None of this is our fault but simply the result of a collective move away from our historical natural, real food diet to a modern way of life that is largely sedentary and involves eating far too much processed food. Combine this with hormones sent haywire by the contents of our food and it is little wonder that many of us struggle with our weight.

Consequently, there has been a flurry of new research into human nutrition and weight loss in recent years, as doctors and scientists try to come up with the magic bullet solution to the galloping rates of global obesity. At the same time, there is much we can learn from our ancestors in terms of healthy eating, so I thought it would be useful to have a brief look here at some of the latest thinking on diets and weight loss, together with some helpful theories from the past.

Carbs – friend and foe?

One aspect of human nutrition that has long puzzled scientists is why various populations who cling to a hunter-gatherer or pastoral lifestyle seem to be in perfect health on diets containing very different types of macronutrient.

For instance, the Masai of East Africa traditionally live almost exclusively on a diet of milk, meat and blood, yet they are extremely lean and seem to be virtually free from any form of heart disease.[1] Similarly, the Turkana people of Kenya consume a predominantly meat-based diet but also avoid any signs of metabolic syndrome or other signs of ill health.[2] There are many other examples of hunter-gatherer societies (such as the Inuit and the native American Plains Indians of the 19th Century) who have existed quite happily for generations on a diet of just meat and fat, whilst maintaining perfect health. However, numerous other non–

Western groups, including the much-studied Kitavans of Papua New Guinea,[3] live on a diet that is almost exclusively carbohydrate, whilst also remaining remarkably healthy.

Carbohydrates are made from sugar, so how can a high carbohydrate diet be healthy? All these people take fairly high levels of daily activity, so are we just back to calories in – calories out again? Not necessarily – virtually all these disparate groups will get fat and succumb to modern diseases if and when they are exposed to our Western diet.[4] In fact, they appear to suffer much more in terms of sudden onset obesity and Type 2 diabetes when exposed to a Western diet, compared to those of us of European origin who have lived on the Western diet since birth.[5,6] So, the key seems to be that something in our diet is upsetting both our bodies and those of non-Western peoples when they abandon their traditional way of eating.

Carbohydrate intolerance

We know that processed carbohydrates (sugar) contain loads of calories and play havoc with our insulin/glucagon system, leading directly to weight gain. However, this is just one example of the numerous damaging effects of our modern diet. In reality, most of us are basically allergic to modern, processed foods, such that we find it very difficult to digest these foods without making ourselves ill and/or fat.

The term 'carbohydrate intolerance' has been coined to explain our inability to properly digest the high sugar foods of our modern diet.[7] This is why I quite understand why many nutritionists and diet authors promote a low-carb diet – surely, if carbs make us ill (and obese), it makes sense to remove them from our diet? In terms of *processed* carbohydrate and other sources of sugar, I entirely agree. However, the danger is that all carbohydrates have become tarred with the same brush.

The Kitavans – the healthiest people on Earth?

The Kitavans are a traditional people who live as subsistence farmers on Papua New Guinea and are thought to be some of the healthiest people on Earth. Most of their food consists of unprocessed carbohydrate in the form of fresh fruit and vegetables (especially root vegetables), together with limited amounts of meat and fish. What is obvious about these remarkable people is that they have historically had no exposure to modern, processed food – no grains or flour, no sugar and no nasty man-made oils or fats. In summary, the Kitavans, much like the Masai, the Turkana and most of the other aboriginal peoples around the world, eat only natural, unprocessed food.

The low-carbohydrate density of real plant food

How can these people exhibit such astonishing health on a diet that is *high* in carbohydrate? Isn't too much carbohydrate in the diet a very bad thing? We might think so but we would be wrong. The answer is complex but hinges on something known as 'carbohydrate density'.[8]

Density is the mass of something divided by its volume. That's a very dry and boring scientific way of thinking about density, so imagine instead it is Christmas morning and you have just given your partner a very expensive box of chocolates as a present. However, you are rather miffed to find that the box contains mostly tissue paper and only four individual chocolates. Apart from the fact that you have been ripped off, the density of chocolates in the box could well be described as low, I think.

Imagine instead that your partner has received numerous boxes of chocolates on Christmas morning, all with just four chocolates in each one. He or she opens each box in turn, discards the tissue paper, tips each tray of chocolates into one chocolate box and replaces the lid in satisfaction. Now we have a very high density of chocolates!

What has this got to do with carbohydrate? Plants store carbohydrate in their cells as starch but the density of carbohydrate stored in unprocessed plant food, e.g. fruits, tubers, leaves is really rather low, with a maximum density of about 23% by mass (the remaining 77% is mostly water). This is the equivalent density of our original box of chocolates.

By comparison, the processed carbohydrate that makes up the bulk of our modern diet is the equivalent of all the chocolates tipped into one box on Christmas morning. For instance, the food industry takes the seeds (grain) from wheat and subjects them to intensive processing in order to produce flour on an enormous scale. The milling process disrupts the cell walls of the wheat seed which leads to the carbohydrate in each cell being released and concentrated into a sort of 'supercharged' high-density (and high-calorie) carbohydrate product called flour. As we know, this is then turned into lots of naughty foods such as bread, cakes, pasta etc. Interestingly, carbohydrate density does not change during the cooking of real food, as the carbohydrate stays trapped inside the cell with only the joints between the cells themselves broken during the cooking process.

The Kitavans actually eat a healthy, natural plant-based diet

The Kitavans might appear to eat a high-carbohydrate diet with impunity but they eat natural, unprocessed plant foods with a *low* carbohydrate density. Such foods are highly nutritious but contain relatively few calories; the sugar content of their food is very low too, with all the intendent health benefits already discussed. The Kitavans are active all day long and as they eat virtually no processed food, they have a limited insulin response to their diet so remain acutely insulin sensitive as well. This probably explains why they have remarkably low rates of obesity and low markers for many Western diseases, such as heart disease and diabetes.[9]

What, then, makes our typical high-sugar Western diet, based on processed grains, added sugar and 'bad fats', so damaging to our health? The answer is complex and not at all obvious but a key factor appears to be the millions of bacteria living in our gut.

Our gut bacteria might hold sway over our weight

The bacteria that live in our gut and the use of pro and prebiotics to encourage the growth of 'good' gut bacteria is all the rage these days. Once thought of as out of sight and out of mind, such helpful bacteria now appear vital to our overall health and seem able to relieve many of the unpleasant symptoms of our modern diet, such as IBS. However, it is the balance of bacteria in our guts, often disturbed by our modern diet, which might be a key factor in deciding whether or not we will gain weight.[10]

Many bacteria are classed as Gram Negative and have something called bacterial lipopolysaccharide (LPS) in their cell walls. Remarkably, it seems that high levels of LPS from 'bad' bacteria may actually lead directly to obesity.

We humans, including the bacterial passengers inside our guts, evolved over millions of years under a dietary regime of real, unprocessed foods and virtually no sugar. This lack of sugar in the ancestral diet favoured a particular type of gut bacteria, which are helpful to us and form an important part of our digestive and immune systems. However, our modern, high-sugar diet now favours different forms of bacteria that would not have been able to establish a foothold in our guts if we had continued to eat the food we are supposed to eat. Instead, these 'bad' bacteria now flourish and in evolutionary terms, they outcompete the good bacteria for space in our guts. Subsequently, the LPS of these undesirable bacterial interlopers causes inflammation inside us, leading directly to obesity.[11]

Inflammation – a key cause of obesity

When we injure ourselves, the area around the wound becomes red and inflamed, which is just our immune system doing its job in fighting off infection. However, this sort of inflammation happens inside our body as well, especially if we eat a high-sugar diet. Too much sugar feeds the bad bacteria and so upsets the balance of the bugs in our guts, particularly in the small intestine. This means we end up with increased numbers of bad LPS circulating around our bodies, which in turn sets up an inflammatory response that leads directly to a number of health problems, such as increased risk of heart disease or cancer. Unfortunately, this sort of internal inflammation can also make us resistant to both insulin and leptin. And as we know, this sort of hormonal resistance lies at the heart of the obesity issue.

New thoughts on ancient foods – the Mediterranean diet

The Mediterranean diet is a rather general term used to sum up the diet of people in the Mediterranean region going back thousands of years.[12] In scientific terms, the Mediterranean diet refers mainly to the diet and lifestyle of subsistence farmers on the island of Crete in the mid-twentieth century. This is due to a famous research project started in the 1950s by Ancel Keys, known as the Seven Countries Study.[13]

It is difficult to come up with a straightforward

definition of what exactly constitutes the Mediterranean diet, as the specifics of what people eat now (or more accurately, ate in the past) vary from country to country around the Mediterranean region. Nevertheless, most scientists agree that a true Mediterranean diet consists of high levels of plant foods (mostly fruits, salad plants, herbs and vegetables that would have been traditionally grown or gathered from the local fields and hillsides), together with plentiful legumes, some rough bread, a little cheese, quite a lot of fish and perhaps meat only a few times a year on high days and holidays.[14] The main fat source is from virgin olive oil (as much as 40% of calories consumed in Greece) and from the fish. Red wine seems to accompany every meal! A true Mediterranean diet does *not* contain the more harmful foods typical of our modern Western diet, e.g. highly processed carbohydrate foods, sugars, trans fats, processed meats.

Compared to modern foods that are high in calories, sugars and modified fats, a true Mediterranean diet is a healthy and beneficial way to eat.[15] More specifically, there is growing evidence that a Mediterranean diet can prevent cardiovascular disease and may well be effective in preventing or reversing metabolic syndrome, fighting cancer and extending lifespan.[16,17] Of particular interest are the recent findings that show how a Mediterranean diet can help in the fight against weight gain and obesity, too.[18,19]

There is also a growing awareness of the health benefits of virgin olive oil, now my favoured dietary fat.[20,21] A typical Mediterranean diet also features a fair amount of bread but I think we would be generally better off giving wheat products a wide berth as much as possible. The current scientific evidence supports this view, too.[22]

First and foremost, a true Mediterranean diet is a *plant-based diet*, not a diet heavy in meat and other animal products. Such plant foods are in their natural state and not heavily processed. The Mediterranean diet is as close to a Back to Basics diet as makes no odds, so I highly recommend adding some onion, garlic, virgin olive oil, fresh fish, lots of salads and vegetables (and of course, a little red wine on the side) to the Back to Basics meal plans. On a hot sunny day, we might even close our eyes and imagine we are sitting barefoot at a beachside taverna by a wine-dark sea…

Going the whole hog – a complete plant-based diet for weight loss?

Humans have been eating animals for millions of years but it is hard to ignore the clamour these days (from many different quarters) for the adoption of a complete plant-based (vegan) diet.[23–26] Could a *completely* plant-based diet be a natural human diet? Regardless of the ethical concerns as to our right to eat animals (more later), in pure nutritional terms, is a *complete* plant-based diet better for weight loss and improved health compared to a Back to Basics, *predominantly* plant-based diet?

A pure plant diet *might* be more effective in achieving weight loss when compared to a non-vegetarian diet.[27,28] Similarly, new research has thrown a spotlight on the potential ability of a complete (sometimes low-fat) plant diet to improve Type 2 diabetes, reduce inflammation via the gut microbiota and otherwise provide a holistic boost to health.[29–31] Researchers do caution that any pure plant diet might require supplementation with certain vitamins and minerals, ideally from dietary sources.[32]

Where does this leave those of us who want to eat animal foods now and again? Well, I don't think the occasional piece of chicken or fish is going to do us any harm. Apart from the fact we humans evolved to eat a certain amount of animal foods, it is much easier to put together a healthy way of eating that includes some animal foods, rather than trying to go 100% plant-based straightaway. This is why I favour a *predominantly* plant-based diet, rather than forcing the issue with a pure plant diet.

Nevertheless, any discussion about 100% plant diets must also consider the ethical question of whether or not we have the right to eat animals at all in this day and age. If we are honest, few of us have probably given more than a passing thought as to where our food comes from or the farming practices that are involved in putting such food on the table. That's before we even consider the wider picture of how our food choices impact the environment or affect climate change, for instance.

This all forms a preamble to the question: "Could I eat in a way that enables me to lose weight and improve my health whilst at the same time making room for environmental and animal welfare issues as well?" I think the answer is definitely 'yes' but in suggesting an answer to this complex issue by way of a 100% plant-based diet, I will very quickly find myself in deep water regarding personal choices, ethics, the whys and wherefores of animal husbandry and the whole thorny subject of whether or not we have the right to eat animals at all.

So, whilst I think we should all consider these issues carefully and come up with our own decisions, any further discussion of these matters lies outside the remit of this book. From a purely health point of view, a 100% plant-based diet *may* be the healthiest diet any of us could ever eat. However, eating some animal foods allows us to gain a good source of protein and certainly makes things easier in terms of creating a dietary template to follow for the rest of our lives. Whether we should be eating animals at all is a whole different question and one that only we can answer on our own. And I will leave it at that.

8

Breaking old habits

One of the most daunting aspects of changing our relationship with food and embracing a healthy lifestyle is the thought of having to break the habits of a lifetime. We all have our own vices and comforts in life and it can sometimes seem impossible to envisage a future in which such comforts no longer exist. Nevertheless, to make all this work, we have to face up to our demons and accept that we are going to have to make some big changes.

They say 'it only takes twenty-one days to change a habit' and that may be so, but I think we should probably invest a bit more time and effort in adjusting to a new healthy diet and lifestyle. This is where the Back to Basics diet comes in – by providing a template for changing to a whole new way of eating and getting active, we no longer need to dwell on the bad habits of our past. Instead, we can focus on weight loss in the short term before using the system as a lifelong framework for maintaining health and a perfect weight in the years ahead.

Willpower? Not needed here

We all know how hard it is to stick to a traditional diet. We begin full of good intentions, only to find after a couple of weeks that the wheels fall off and we return to the comfort of our old ways. You and I are not alone – millions of well-intentioned people fall off the diet wagon every year, even though they are just as desperate to lose weight as we are. The problem on most diets is that we are expected to eat very small portions of food to achieve any sort of weight loss, which means having to use huge amounts of willpower just to resist eating more food. We will certainly lose weight in the short term but because the meals are so small, we will soon get hungry and no amount of willpower will resist our urge to eat. If the diet also involves weird, expensive or obscure ingredients, it is highly unlikely that we will stick with it for any length of time, either.

Despite the plethora of fad diets that exist today, any form of food restriction is doomed to failure because we can never resist our innate desire to eat. Somehow though, we have to reduce how many calories we eat, which is where the plant-based diet comes in. By basing our meals around large portions of vegetables, certain grains and legumes, salads and fruits, we can fill ourselves up, reduce the calories and get vastly more micronutrients (vitamins, minerals, phytonutrients etc) than we may have had in a long time. We will finally be in control of our appetites and no longer crying out for nutrients, meaning we won't need to rely on will power all the time to stop us reaching for the biscuit tin. The beauty of filling up with healthy, nutritious plant food is that we simply won't feel hungry; in fact, much of our 'hunger' is just sugar and micronutrient cravings, neither of which is ever truly satisfied with a high-calorie, low-nutrient modern diet.

Using willpower to make changes

The only willpower we need to use is in making the change to a new way of eating and a new lifestyle. We just need to take that first step to *changing*; changing how we eat, changing and organizing our daily routine, changing our shopping habits and changing our whole life by committing, really committing, to following the plan. We will then be off and running – our cravings will ease and we will not require any more willpower to stick to the programme for the rest of our lives.

Getting active every day

As well as changing what and when we eat, to lose weight and improve our health we are going to have to take some exercise as well. The good news is that from now on, I will use the much more friendly term 'activity'. Getting active every day is central to the Back to Basics diet, so it is time to face those demons and accept that we need to break one of our most ingrained habits, the habit of being sedentary.

Understandably, most of us have lost sight of what constitutes normal levels of human activity, i.e. the level of exercise you and I are designed, by evolution, to take. This is certainly the case if we compare the amount of activity we take in our day-to-day lives to how active our Stone Age ancestors were, or how active any number of aboriginal peoples or subsistence farmers around the world are today.

What is the best form of activity? It's called Life

As nutrition blogger Stephan Guyenet once said, "Our ancestors had a different word for exercise – Life!" This sums up our problem in a nutshell; from our hunter-gatherer ancestors right through to the subsistence farmers on the Island of Crete in the 1950s, life was characterized by almost constant activity, often involving hard physical effort and manual labour in just about every waking hour. Not only did these people burn oodles of calories but they also developed healthy, strong bodies, too.

So, where does our twice-weekly trip to the spinning class at the gym fit into this story? Well, it is certainly better than nothing. Nevertheless, if we then spend the rest of the week doing no exercise at all, we are not really making any difference to our long-term health. Instead, we need to take some tips from these more traditional peoples and try to change our whole attitude to activity on a daily basis.

Learning to walk all over again

It seems our earliest ancestors did not suffer from obesity or many other modern diseases, such as cancer, heart disease etc. To be blunt, fat people would not have survived for long in those days because they would have literally fallen by the wayside and been left for dead. So, how did they stay slim? We know they ate a diet of real, unprocessed, mostly plant foods, supplemented by infrequent meals of meat or fish (including fat, of course) but they were also constantly active.

Did our ancestors have annual gym membership? Did the Neanderthals invent Lycra®? Of course not – they stayed slim because they ate relatively few calories and walked, a lot.

Back in our hunter-gatherer past, every waking moment would have been taken up with a list of simple priorities – find water, find food, find shelter, stay alive and reproduce. Life wasn't terribly complicated in those days. All of this involved a lot of walking (well, perhaps not reproduction!) because every calorie was precious. Daily life was measured in costs; costs in foraging for food, costs in time, costs in risking being eaten by a predator, costs in being attacked by another tribe etc. Our ancestors would not have spent all day running everywhere because that would have used up too many calories. They would have pursued game for extended periods but would have walked for most of the time and perhaps sprinted a few hundred yards for the kill. Similarly, they would have walked until attacked by a predator, when they would have again sprinted to get away before dropping back later to a walk once again. Calories had to be preserved at all costs. The walking would have kept them very fit and without the damage to their joints that can occur from too much jogging. Food was scarce and although these people might have appeared very lean, they would have had enough body fat to see them through periods of famine.

We are designed to walk

There is little doubt that we are meant to walk. In fact, one of the most important changes that happened in our evolution from ape to Man was when we stood up and started to walk on our hind legs. Walking requires no special equipment and can be easily included in our daily lives. Walking is fun, either on our own or in the company of friends and family. I think the fitness professionals suggest we keep to a pace that allows us to hold a conversation. I love walking and just enjoy being outside, feeling the sun (or wind and rain where I live) on my face. It's best to avoid busy main roads and remote parks after dark but we need to start getting active every single day and the easiest way to do this is to walk as much as we can. Together with a real food, plant-based Back to Basics diet, daily walking is a really big help in making lifelong improvements to our health.

For those who prefer to cycle, by all means get on your bike instead. If you like swimming then please go swimming whenever you can. All that matters is that we get active every day and the easiest way to do this is to build activity into our day. Here are some suggestions for how we can build activity into each and every day:

GETTING ACTIVE EVERY DAY

- Catch the bus to work? Walk instead.
- Pushed for time? Walk to the bus stop a mile down the road, not the one outside your front door.
- Walk the kids to school and back home again in the afternoon.
- Go for a walk around the park at lunchtime, rather than

sitting idly in the staff canteen stuffing our faces with processed food. ☺
- Take the kids for a walk around the park after school or get a dog and walk him twice a day, every day.
- Have to be in the office by 9.00 am? Set your alarm an hour earlier and cycle to work, rather than using the car. Obviously, you have to cycle home at the end of the day.
- Join a walking/cycling club, go hiking in the hills at weekends, go for a walk before getting the kids ready for school, go out for a bike ride for pleasure etc.
- Find something that suits – staying on the couch is not an option.

Although we all go about our lives in a similar way, we all have different priorities and personal circumstances. We just need to look at our own daily routine to find ways to build activity into our new, healthy lifestyle.

Are you still too busy?

We can all come up with excuses as to why we can't find time to get active: "But I'm too busy to exercise, I've got a business to run. It's a nightmare to get the kids ready for school, I have to go to work, do the shopping AND cook the dinner…" We are all busy but as I said earlier, unless we put *our* health and happiness first, nothing will change. We have to make some time for ourselves and part of that is working out how we can get active every day. It does take a bit of planning and reorganization but will soon become routine (and fun). Later, we can invite our family and friends to join in and get active, too. For now though, we need to find a way to get active every day.

Taking things further

If you want to take things further, there is plenty of help out there in the form of websites, gyms, personal trainers etc. However, for those who haven't done any exercise for a long time, it is just sensible to start off nice and slow by getting out of the house and walking in the first instance. This will make a huge difference to our ability to burn fat and lose weight compared to steadfastly remaining on the couch.

Nevertheless, if the exercise bug takes hold, get a bicycle, take up a sport, learn a martial art, go swimming or play tennis – we just need to be careful not to overdo it in the early weeks and months of our new regime. For those who are very heavy or otherwise new to any form of activity, have a medical check-up first and then just stick to walking for the time being, certainly until some weight has been lost and a basic level of fitness has been achieved.

Daily activity helps but eating right is the key to weight loss

At the beginning of the book, I explained that to lose weight we had to consume fewer calories than we burn up. The Back to Basics diet helps with this because the foods I recommend are naturally low in calories. Although getting active is hugely important in improving our health and wellbeing, permanent weight loss and improved health are mostly down to what (and when) we eat. Nevertheless, it would make life much easier if we could work on the other side of the 'calories in– calories out' equation, too. Our Basal Metabolic Rate (BMR) gives us the number of calories we need to stay alive under normal conditions (see Appendix 1 for BMR sum). The recommended eating plans in this programme make it hard to eat much more than our BMR each day but any activity we can do above and beyond our BMR will tip the 'calories in–calories out' equation in our favour. If we burn up more calories than we eat our body will have to find those extra calories from our stores of glycogen and fat. And if we can minimize the time we spend insulinated by daily fasting, we will make it much easier for our body to access this fat as well.

Using a heart rate monitor to see those calories disappear

A great aid for getting active is something called a heart rate monitor. This is just a simple and relatively cheap piece of sports equipment that one can buy at most sports shops or online for about £30 or thereabouts. They need a bit of setting up to begin with (inputting age, sex, weight etc) and after that, the brain in the monitor does the rest. Basically, this clever gadget records heart rate very accurately and as you start to huff and puff, it calculates how many calories you are using, as well as keeping track of time, training zones, heart rate etc. One useful tip is to wear the monitor to work now and again. It is very discreet under clothes, so nobody will know! Have a go then at an all-day workout, e.g. walk to work, use the stairs not the lift, stand up as much as possible during the day, go for a walk at lunchtime, walk up and down a few more flights of stairs and walk home at the end of the day. The heart rate monitor will tell you how many calories you have burned, so you can easily adjust and tweak your daily activity to burn more and more calories each day. A heart rate monitor is a very useful device and well worth the investment.

9

Summing it all up

It always seems impossible until it's done.
Nelson Mandela

For many years, people around the world have been moving from the farmlands to towns and cities in search of a better life and higher wages. This has led to a complete change in the way we eat. Having left the world of subsistence agriculture behind, food now has to be produced on a massive scale, requiring a level of food processing never before seen in human history. On top of that, we have also been told for decades to eat a 'low-fat diet', advice that has quite possibly been the single biggest factor behind the pandemic of obesity we see today.

Moreover, since the 1960s or thereabouts, we have seen an explosive growth in the fast food culture and simultaneous breakdown in traditional real food meals at home. Add all this together and we have a modern global society that perceives normal eating as the constant grazing of calorie-rich but nutritionally poor processed (mostly carbohydrate) foods, coupled to reduced levels of activity. This all leads to a massive intake of calories, insulin resistance and a worldwide epidemic of obesity and associated diseases, such as Type 2 diabetes.

Our modern diet – the conveyor belt to obesity

The reason so many of us struggle with our weight is due to some dastardly combination of eating the wrong types of foods, eating too many calories, developing internal inflammation and insulin resistance and not taking enough activity! Frankly though, none of this really matters. Let the doctors and scientists argue over the technical pathways that link our modern diet to obesity – all we need to understand is that our old diet of processed carbs, too much trans fat and sugar (Fig 11) not only gave us too many calories for little benefit but also upset our body chemistry such that it was almost impossible to resist putting on weight. This is why I say it is not our fault that we put on weight these days.

Our weight is ultimately controlled by how many calories we eat, compared to the calories we use up each day of our lives. Nevertheless, the advice to simply 'eat less and move more' will never work unless we take a root-and-branch look at our diet and lifestyle, as we have done here in *The Back to Basics Diet*. We have gone to great lengths to work out why we get fat, why being overweight is bad for our health, why we tend to eat too many calories these days and why the modern, processed foods we are surrounded by cause us to switch over to storing, not burning, fat. Simply trying to eat less (modern) food will never address any of these issues. Instead, the secret to healthy, lifelong weight loss involves eating fewer calories via a natural, real food, plant-based diet that also supplies us with plentiful nutrients for relatively few calories and at the same time gives our hormones a rest.

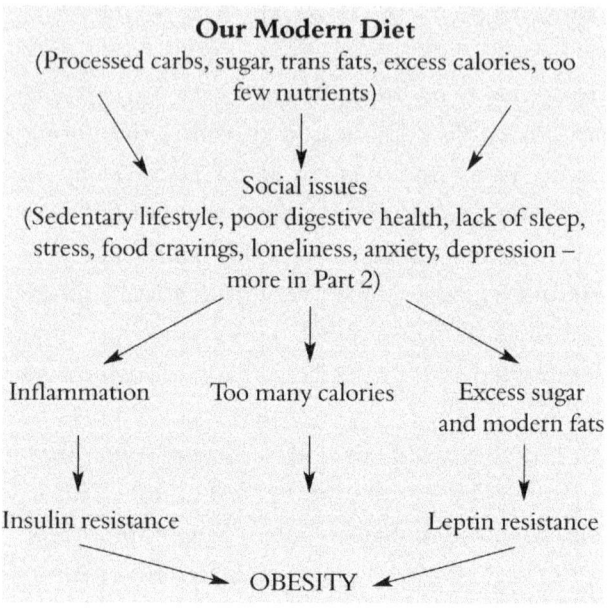

Fig 11. Our modern diet – the root cause of our obesity

By getting back to basics and truly changing what and when we eat, our obesity will eventually be banished forever. Our insulin sensitivity should also improve, such that we give ourselves the best chance of avoiding Type 2 diabetes in future. Best of all, just being on the journey to a correct weight and much-improved health is inspiring and empowering, such that life no longer seems so overwhelming and we can again discover our self-esteem. Life is something to cherish and enjoy and as I am constantly reminded, not a rehearsal; so let's lose weight, get fit and enjoy every day.

See you in Part 2.

PART TWO

The Back to Basics Diet

10

Seven weeks to change your life

The journey of a thousand miles begins with one step.
Lao Tzu

It is now time to put the theory into practice, which is why here in Part 2 you will find all the information needed to get your weight loss underway. This includes the Back to Basics diet plans themselves (together with a detailed explanation as to how they work) plus the initial seven-week transition plan as well.

The Back to Basics diet is not a quick fix or crash diet but a programme for life. The initial seven-week programme gets things underway, where hopefully the diet plan(s) and accompanying recipes will help you think about food in a new and mindful way. This includes what and when to eat, how to shop and how to prepare simple meals in line with the Back to Basics philosophy. Later, the Maintenance Programme provides a follow-on to the Basic Programme and is an ideal way to keep on the straight and narrow in the months and years ahead. This way, the Back to Basics diet becomes a template for making the right food and activity choices for the rest of our lives.

Everything that follows is designed to make life as

simple as possible in terms of deciding *what* and *when* to eat. This will soon become second nature, so life can continue without us having to constantly fret over what to eat or how that affects our weight and long-term health. The most important task in the early stages is to get rid of the processed, sugary junk; after that, start getting used to eating a healthy, real food diet and try to get active every day. Having picked one of the two Back to Basics diet programmes, read through it a couple of times, get organized with the shopping and the cooking and just follow it day by day.

Seven weeks to change your life

To help transition to a plant-based, real food diet and healthy lifestyle, it helps to start one day at a time. As there are seven days in the week, it makes sense to use that to our advantage by taking seven weeks to complete the transition to a Back to Basics way of life. Therefore, in Week One, follow the Back to Basics programme to the letter on one day that week. Choose your preferred diet plan and whichever day of the week you wish to start, then simply choose a day from the plan to follow for that day. In Week Two, follow the programme for two days that week and so on. After seven weeks, you will have completed the transition to the Back to Basics programme in nice, easy stages. This simple seven-week programme is summarized here:

The Back to Basics seven-week diet programme

Weeks	Follow the Back to Basics programme on:
Week One	*One day*
Week Two	*Two days*
Week Three	*Three days*
Week Four	*Four days*
Week Five	*Five days*
Week Six	*Six days*
Week Seven	*All week!*

Once you have reached week seven, just stick with your chosen plan until you have lost sufficient weight or are otherwise comfortable to move on to the maintenance programme. The rate of weight loss might slow a bit on the maintenance programme but you can always return to the diet plan for a week or two if you so wish. Nevertheless, this new way of eating and getting active every day has life-changing benefits above and beyond the fixation we all have with our waistlines. The last few pounds will soon disappear (even on the Maintenance Programme), so we can relax knowing that we are continuing to feed our bodies a fantastic low-calorie, nutrient-rich diet.

There are some recipes at the end of the book, which I hope will be helpful. However, please feel free to research your own recipes and new ways to be active every day as well. Each plan contains a two-week template with daily food and activity suggestions, which can be followed to the letter or tweaked to suit your own tastes. In the future, if you have a wobble or just want someone else to do the thinking for you for a while, come back to the programme and follow it closely until you are happy to go solo once more. The Back to Basics diet, full of health-giving nutrients but relatively few calories, is simple, straightforward and easy to follow, both in the short term and in the years ahead.

The Back to Basics diet plans

There is a choice of plans on the Back to Basics programme. The main plan is the Basic Programme, whilst the Modified Programme is aimed at those who are unable to exercise due to injury or disability. Each plan combines healthy meal choices, alteration to meal timings and daily activity into one, holistic system that can be followed for as long as you like. No tricks, no gimmicks, just eating in accordance with our evolutionary design. Each plan has been designed around the main principles of this book, e.g. the use of intermittent fasting to minimize the time spent insulinated (making best use of low insulin levels to access fat reserves) and daily activity to really burn off the fat, once and for all.

Each Back to Basics diet plan contains the following types and quantities of foods:

- Real, natural foods that provide high levels of nutrients for low amounts of calories. Meals are based around fruit, salads and vegetables, all of which are relatively energy-poor (low in calories) but nutrient-rich, i.e. full of phytochemicals, vitamins, anti-oxidants, proteins, healthy fats and carbohydrates that are essential for health.

- 80%–90% of each meal should comprise high-quality (preferably organic) vegetables and fruit. Green vegetables and wild fruits, e.g. berries are the panacea to good health.

- The remainder of the diet (10–20%) should be high-quality protein from vegetables, legumes, fish, poultry, lean meat, eggs, nuts etc and healthy fats.

- If you must eat red meat, eat it rarely and make sure it is organic or wild game.

- Use organic olive oil or a balanced Omega 6 : Omega 3 oil, such as Udo's Oil, as a primary fat source – flaxseed is good, too.

- We should all watch our alcohol intake but the odd glass of wine is perfectly OK. If you are really struggling, an occasional baked potato, single piece of wholemeal bread or small portion of brown rice is fine, once in a while.

Quantities of food

I haven't mentioned portion size much so far as I think it is more important to concentrate on the types of food we eat, rather than fixate on portion control. Nevertheless, I think sensible portion control just means eating until we are pleasantly replete, not completely stuffed. By eating a plant-based, real food diet, the calories will largely take care of themselves, so it is quite normal to eat a big portion of food at each mealtime. This is one of the key factors of the Back to Basics diet – no tiny portions of food here! If you want more guidance on portion size, try eating no more food at each meal than would fill a normal-sized dessert bowl or dinner plate.

Timings of meals and snacks

Meals on the Back to Basics diet are timed to maximize the low-insulin phases of the day, i.e. eat as late as possible in the morning, after we have taken our morning activity, and eat early in the evening after another bout of activity. This way, you spend much more time primed to burn fat, not store fat. Ideally, the first meal of the day should be eaten as late in the morning as possible. At the very least, try to do some activity before eating breakfast. Eventually, try to squeeze all meals into a small segment of the day e.g. brunch/early lunch around midday, afternoon snack and early evening meal. If really hungry, have another snack of fruit or raw veggies or in extremis, another small real food meal. However, we shouldn't ever get truly hungry as we will be eating plenty of food (at similar times each day), which will help our system settle down and so relieve those dreaded hunger pangs.

Treats

We all like a food treat occasionally but we must be careful not to view a bit of naughty food or 'just one more glass of wine' as an excuse for not fully committing to a healthy diet and lifestyle. We might suffer the odd craving at first but these will soon disappear once the change is made from a sugar-laden, low-nutrient diet to a healthy, high-nutrient diet instead. A tip I picked up somewhere is when cravings strike, drink a glass of water. In extremis, go out for a walk. It really works. On a serious note, it is quite common to have genuine addictions to certain foods, addictions that can be as difficult to break as those involving alcohol, tobacco or recreational drugs. For anyone in that category, I strongly recommend seeking out professional help; I sought help myself in the past and it changed my life. I will talk about treats in a bit more detail in the next chapter, under the heading *identifying addiction triggers* but in the meantime, if you can stop smoking and get off (most) of the booze, you will go a long way to boosting your self-esteem and make your diet and lifestyle reboot much easier as well.

Activity

We need to try to get active every day if at all possible, which is why I recommend walking a little each day in the first instance. If you are very heavy and/or very unfit, have a chat with your doctor before you start. Save up and buy a heart rate monitor and some trainers because it will make all the difference. Go outside and get active in the morning (make it part of your journey to work, for instance) and try to go for another walk before you sit down to your evening meal. Don't worry about what other people think – just get out of that front door. Here are some other activity suggestions:

- Walk or cycle to work
- Walk the kids to school and back home again in the afternoon
- Cycle with the kids to school
- Get a dog – no excuses for not walking then!
- Go swimming
- Join a gym if you wish, but not necessary in the early stages
- Dance round the house to music
- Use a TV fitness programme
- Take up a sport
- Take up a martial art
- Dig the garden

Try to make some sort of activity part of daily life. It is amazing how empowering it is to get outside every day and take some form of exercise; very soon, you won't believe how you could have lived for so long without being active.

Falling off the wagon

The diet and lifestyle changes in the Back to Basics diet may seem daunting at first but they are actually very straightforward and will soon become second nature once you have completed the initial seven-week programme. Nevertheless, there are bound to be a few hiccups along the way, so please don't worry too much if you have the occasional wobble. It happens to us all at times, so just pick yourself up and carry on with the programme – you'll get there in the end. Be mindful and remember why you are trying to change. It is time to look after Number One; everything has to come second to that, just for a while.

Stop, Breathe, Think, Act

None of us is naturally selfish and we have probably spent a lifetime looking after our partners, our children and our friends and family before thinking about our needs at all. However, if we are not mindful of our own needs, it is easy to be lulled into temptation when we are 'elsewhere', i.e. thinking about all the other people who depend on us. So, to help stay focused in the face of temptation, here is a tip I picked up from a completely different part of my life (scuba diving, actually) that works brilliantly in the context of sticking to changes in the diet. The next time temptation strikes (in the form of a sandwich, a piece of toast or a cream bun), just stop for a moment, take a deep breath, think about what you are doing and turn away. It only takes a second but being mindful in this way can help us avoid ordering that sandwich or picking up a packet of biscuits at the petrol station purely out of habit. This is just another way to reboot our behaviour around food, that's all.

Choosing your Back to Basics diet plan

The Back to Basics diet plans follow in the next chapter; please choose whichever one best suits your personal circumstances. Each plan provides a daily programme to follow to help you on your way to a healthy weight. After the initial seven-week phase, just stick with your particular plan for as long as you wish until ready to switch over to the Maintenance Programme; this is a slightly modified version of the Back to Basics diet designed to act as a general guide to what and when to eat (and when to get active) in the years ahead. Have a look at each plan in turn and choose one to get started. Most of us should stick with the Basic Programme but whichever plan you choose, you will find a template of meals and activity and detailed advice as to how to structure your day around a healthy eating and activity regime.

11

The Back to Basics Diet Programmes

I can resist everything except temptation.
Oscar Wilde

Welcome to the Back to Basics diet programmes, the foundation of the Back to Basics diet. The Basic Programme is at the core of the Back to Basics diet and includes daily activity, whilst the Modified Programme is designed for those who, for whatever reason, are unable to exercise. Please choose whichever programme suits you best. Once you have made your choice, use the seven-week system to transition over to a real food, plant-based diet, for life.

Each programme provides a framework of meals (and daily activity on the Basic Programme) to help get your weight loss journey underway. There are some tips and tricks and 'rules of the game' as well, which follow after the programme descriptions. Finally, there is a Maintenance Programme to follow in the months and years ahead.

This is not a quick fix or another fad diet. Instead, the Back to Basics diet is designed to help make significant changes to your diet and lifestyle to ensure you can lose weight, improve your health and fitness and stop the weight yo-yoing that is so common with traditional diets.

Choosing a programme

The Basic Programme includes daily activity, so should be the choice for most of us. However, for those who are infirm or otherwise unable to exercise, the modified version instead restricts calories through strict portion control. Later, the Maintenance Programme serves to keep us on the straight and narrow once we are comfortable with the diet programme and have lost sufficient weight.

Getting organized

It is well worth spending a few minutes with pen and paper before getting underway with the programme, just to do a little planning. For instance, which day of the week do you want to start your seven-week initial phase? Which meals/recipes do you want to try? What do you need to buy to stock up your store cupboard? Just give yourself the time to think about these sorts of questions before you start.

Identifying addiction triggers

Many of us have a soft spot for certain types of food or drink, the comforts we turn to when we are fed up or depressed. This is not something to be embarrassed about but it makes sense to identify such foods, so that we can either get rid of them completely or at least restrict the times we have access to them. If we can identify the foods that may have led us to put on weight, we can replace them with healthier versions when we need a comfort. This is much easier than trying to banish comfort eating completely – an apple, handful of nuts or some crudités and hummus is a much better option than reaching for a cake or the biscuit tin. If the sweet tooth is acting up, try eating a piece of fruit, not a chocolate biscuit. If feeling peckish, drink a glass of water or walk around the block. If that doesn't work, eat some fruit, nuts, raw veggies or a piece of protein, e.g. some cold chicken, for instance. It is all about the big picture – we are trying to change the (bad) habits of a lifetime, so everything we can do to give ourselves the best chance of success, the easier life will become.

Go shopping

This is where a bit of planning comes in handy, e.g. can I get everything I need at the local supermarket or will I have to widen the net? We want the real foods we looked at in Chapter 4, so mostly fruit and vegetables, some fish, some poultry perhaps, herbs, spices, some olive oil maybe, that sort of thing. None of this need be expensive; I have found I spend less money on food now than I did in when I bought loads of junk and alcohol, for instance. Try the local farmers' market or perhaps use a box scheme to get organic veggies and fruit delivered to your door. Can you grow your own? It also helps to have a good look around the local supermarket; what is their fruit and veg like, how expensive is it compared to the other supermarket down the road, how much organic produce do they have? Do you want to go shopping every couple of days or would you rather get a home delivery? Thinking about how to source real foods in this way puts us front and centre in all decisions regarding our new diet, which in itself makes shopping for real foods as important a part of re-establishing a healthy relationship with food as what we eat for dinner each day.

Give it a go

Once you are ready and the fridge is stocked with fresh fruits, salads, vegetables and healthy proteins, just give it a go. Use the seven-week step-by-step system (below) to transition over to a Back to Basics way of life. Simply choose a day to follow from your chosen plan and stick to it for one day in the first week. In Week Two, follow the programme for two days a week and so on. After seven weeks, you will have completed the transition to the Back to Basics programme, in nice, easy stages.

Weeks	Follow the Back to Basics programme on:
Week One	*One day*
Week Two	*Two days*
Week Three	*Three days*
Week Four	*Four days*
Week Five	*Five days*
Week Six	*Six days*
Week Seven	*All week!*

I'm sure you will love it and won't look back once you get started. Good luck.

The Back to Basics Basic Programme

- Alarm clock goes off. Time to face the world.

- *Get active:* Go for a brisk walk or otherwise do some physical activity, ideally out in the fresh air. Maybe walk or cycle to work or walk the kids to school? Try to be active before eating your breakfast or brunch.

- *Breakfast*: Have a cup of tea or coffee if you want but see if you can hold out till later in the morning before eating. If that's too difficult, just wait until after your morning activity before eating your breakfast.

- *Brunch/Lunch*: Try to make this the first meal of the day. If you eat breakfast, do not eat again until later in the day, i.e. have a late lunch, not a brunch two hours after breakfast. This way, we keep a check on our calorie intake and let insulin levels return to a resting level between meals.

- *Afternoon snack*: Try some fresh fruit or raw veggies with hummus or a handful of nuts.

- *Late afternoon activity*: Try to do some more activity now if possible. Go for another walk or walk/cycle home from work. Play with the kids in the back garden or in the local park. Go to the gym if that suits.

- *Evening meal*: Time for a tasty, nutritious real food, plant-based meal with friends and family. Keep it simple at first – choose a protein (such as fish, chicken, turkey, quinoa, chickpeas etc) and add plenty of veggies or salad. If you suffer from an upset tum now and again, stick to cooked vegetables at first, rather than too much raw plant food. Add spices and flavours as much as you like. Use olive oil or Udo's Oil in moderation for salad dressing and don't worry too much about fat in food otherwise. Enjoy a glass of wine if you wish but have some fresh fruit for pudding, not spotted dick and custard. ☺

- *Time to relax*: Enjoy some quality time with your partner, family, friends etc.

- *Bedtime*: Over to you!

Two weeks on the Back to Basics diet

Basic Programme

What follows is a two-week plan of suggested meals and daily activity built around a structured day on the Basic Programme. Nothing is set in stone, so please use this as a guide and make changes to recipes, meal times and daily routine as necessary.

Once you are comfortable with the programme, have a go at creating your own meals. Keep it simple – there is no need for complex or highfalutin recipes here. Try having a Wonder Salad at each meal, either as a main course or as a side dish. Take it to work, eat it for supper or have it for breakfast. This is a plant-based diet, so eat plenty of green salads and vegetables.

Buy a good quality joint/chicken, make it last two or

three meals, make stock, make soups, grow your own veg etc. Basically, use any combination of healthy protein, i.e. fish, chicken, turkey, eggs, cheese, or vegetable foods like lentils, chickpeas, hummus etc with lots of salad, veggies etc. Red meat is OK in moderation but chicken, fish and vegetable protein are better. Have some berry fruit for dessert (strawberries and cream are great in summer). Eat plenty of food at each meal.

Sample two-week plan on the Back to Basics Basic Programme

Week One	Am activity	Brunch	Snack	Pm activity	Dinner
Monday	Walk, cycle, swim etc	Cold chicken, salad/ veggies	Fresh Fruit	Walk, cycle, swim etc	One-Minute Wonder Salad
Tuesday	"	Tuna salad	Nuts and veggies	"	Home-made soup
Wednesday	"	Omelette and salad	Fresh fruit	"	Smoked haddock and veggies
Thursday	"	Vegetable curry	Fresh fruit	"	Quinoa and salad
Friday	"	Salmon salad	Nuts and veggies	"	Dave's daal and veggies
Saturday	"	Bacon and mushrooms	Crudités and hummus	"	Salade Nicoise
Sunday	"	Sunday roast	Fresh fruit	"	Cold cuts and salad

Week Two	Am activity	Brunch	Snack	Pm activity	Dinner
Monday	Walk, cycle, swim etc	Turkey and avocado salad	Fresh Fruit	Walk, cycle, swim etc	Easy lamb casserole
Tuesday	"	Greek salad	Nuts and veggies	"	Spicy quinoa
Wednesday	"	Chickpea salad	Fresh fruit	"	Quick spicy beef mince and veggies
Thursday	"	Lentil soup	Fresh fruit	"	Simple Moroccan chicken
Friday	"	Back to Basics Buddha bowl	Nuts and veggies	"	Baked salmon
Saturday	"	Baked curry cauliflower	Crudités and hummus	"	Succulent slow roast lamb
Sunday	"	Tender roast pork	Fresh fruit	"	Cold cuts and salad

The recipes for all the meals in the two-week plan (plus others) are in Chapter 13. In addition, I have listed a few other ideas for brunches and dinners below. Once you are comfortable eating this way, feel free to work out your own meal plans and recipes that suit your personal tastes and interests. I've tried to keep things as simple as possible (I'm a man!) and have just listed a few more ideas for brunch or dinner to start the ball rolling. Ideally, eat just two main meals a day. Anyway, here are a few more suggested meals to help you on your way:

Some brunch suggestions
- Berry fruits (strawberries, raspberries, blueberries etc) and goat's yoghurt
- Strawberries and Champagne (wedding anniversary?)
- Scrambled eggs and smoked salmon
- Porridge oats (a bit 'carby' but OK in moderation, if you must)
- Bircher muesli (ditto)
- Dave's kedgeree
- Smoked haddock and poached egg

Some dinner suggestions
- Salad Caprese
- Grilled Mediterranean vegetables, with fish perhaps
- Huge salad plus some chicken, fish, cold meats etc
- Vegetable curry (plus a small portion of organic brown basmati if you wish)
- Vegetable soup
- Healthy chicken and veggie soup
- A One-Minute Wonder Salad plus tuna, cold chicken or roast beef etc
- Gilly's wonderful Asian fish (or similar recipe)
- Quinoa and salad

- Roast chicken plus steamed veggies etc

Off to work?

Here are some ideas for packed brunch and/or lunch:

- Cold chicken plus salad/veggies
- Hard-boiled eggs plus salad/veggies
- Tomatoes, raw carrots, celery etc plus a pot of Hummus, too
- Berries and yoghurt
- Crudités
- Tin of tuna plus salad, raw veggies etc and a little mayo
- Some homemade soup in a flask
- Bring some salad dressing from home (see my vinaigrette recipe) and buy the following from the canteen, staff restaurant, local shop etc: salads, veggies, chicken breast, fish, turkey, ham etc

Here are four tips that I hope will be useful as you start your Back to Basics diet:

Tip number one: Buy and prepare real foods the way our elders used to do

As we develop a healthy relationship with real food, it is worth looking at how our grandparents' or great-grandparents' generation went about feeding themselves and their families. My grandmother grew up in a poor family around the time of the First World War, so had to learn to make ends meet at a young age. Life was hard, particularly during rationing in the aftermath of World War Two. Nevertheless, she managed to feed her family remarkably well during those difficult years.

Most meals were eaten at home as eating out was expensive and normally reserved for special occasions. Food was hard to come by and expensive in real terms, so had to be made to go a long way. Leftovers were used to make healthy, delicious meals often through to midweek and home cooking, preserving and making do was the order of the day. Many families grew their own fruit and vegetables in the garden.

People walked or bicycled to work, as cars were an expensive luxury beyond the means of most. Apart from popping down to the local chippie for a weekly treat of fish and chips, the idea of ordering a takeaway or buying food at the garage or railway station to eat (in public!) would have been unthinkable. Indeed, many of these wise old ladies would not recognize much of the food we eat today as food. They would certainly be appalled at the breakdown in the social structure of mealtimes and the casual, wasteful way we treat food today. Above all, food was cherished and treated with respect. This is a far cry from our modern world where 'food' is everywhere we look 24/7.

Nowadays, we have a wonderful selection of produce available to us all year round in the shops and supermarkets that, in real terms, is cheaper than it has ever been. However, we have allowed our comfortable, modern life to seduce us into lazy and disorganized eating. Casual meals 'on the go' and takeaways have replaced proper meals made from home-cooked, real food. No, Grandma probably didn't have a full-time job but she almost certainly had less money to spend on food than we do and she definitely didn't have a fully stocked supermarket on her doorstep, with amazing produce from all around the world.

So, let's start putting things back together again by using some of the shopping and cooking techniques of the past. This should help us return to a structured way of eating, where we eat the right types of food at the right times of day, i.e. eating properly, in harmony with our evolutionary design, not grazing all day long on processed foods. It will help to save money as well. If we follow the example of this formidable generation, we can learn to organize ourselves effectively and plan what we are going to eat and when we are going to do our food shopping. This will help us break the habit of saying 'I haven't got any food in the house, I'll get a takeaway'. Instead, we can structure a new way of eating around healthy, home-cooked food, just like dear old Grandma.

As an example, here is a sample week's worth of meals, based on Grandma's common-sense approach but updated with foods available to us in the modern world:

- *Sunday* – I love a traditional Sunday lunch or dinner. A typical roast might be a joint of meat, usually beef, pork or lamb but let's have a roast chicken instead. All the main supermarkets offer free-range birds at reasonable prices but an organic chicken from a reputable local supplier (butcher/farmer etc) will be even better, if you can find one. This may cost a bit more but the Sunday roast will form the basis of at least two further meals, so we are saving money in real terms anyway. Roast in the oven as per my recipe and add loads of veggies and salad for a tasty, delicious meal.

- *Monday* – use the leftover chicken today (if you have a big family, you might have to roast two birds on Sunday), plus the chicken carcass itself and some of the unused vegetables. Off to work on Monday? Take some cold chicken with you, perhaps. Otherwise, you can enjoy a cold chicken salad on Monday evening, plus the rest of the vegetables. This will probably cost you less than a pound. Keep the chicken carcass covered in the fridge.

- *Tuesday* – use the chicken carcass as the basis for a stock, throw in some of the remaining vegetables (perhaps add some leeks and turnips) plus some red lentils from the store cupboard for a wonderful soup on Tuesday evening. Have some fresh fruit for dessert. Cost? Another pound.

- *Wednesday* – a mushroom omelette and salad tonight (see recipe section for how to cook the perfect omelette). We can buy six free-range eggs and use three for the omelette and have the rest during the week. A pack of organic mushrooms and a bag of salad and dinner is sorted for a couple of quid. Cooking time is less than ten minutes.

- *Thursday* – how about a vegetable curry? It is too complicated to list the cost of all ingredients (see recipe section) but budget for less than £10 in total.

- *Friday* – finish off the curry, with another salad and yoghurt, perhaps.

- *Saturday* – how about a big salad with some tinned tuna? Or perhaps a meal out? There is a nice French bistro down the road; I would have a Salade Nicoise and a glass of Sancerre. Total cost? No more than a take away and a six-pack of beer.

This is just an example to show that we can eat simply and cheaply for a whole week (whilst following the principles of the book) and still lose weight. I know that junk food is depressingly cheap but it is possible to eat really healthy, tasty food for not a lot of money. We just need a bit of planning and organization.

All these old-fashioned meals are inherently low in calories and contain foods that are either very low on the Glycaemic Index or simply don't register on it at all. There is very little sugar here either and each of these meals would take time to digest and hence have only a slow and minimal effect on our insulin levels, too. Result? We gain loads of healthy nutrients, eat plentiful portions, have no hunger and see steady, permanent weight loss.

Many of us are overweight because eating has become something we fit in around everything else in our lives; eating has become unplanned and disorganized. 'I'm too busy, I'll just grab something on the way home from work' is not the way to re-establish any sort of healthy relationship with food. However, with a bit of planning, we can get the majority of our week's shopping and meal plans worked out over the weekend, when most of us have time to sit down for a few minutes and take charge of our lives. With practice, this will become second nature. By returning to planning and preparing meals of real foods like Grandma, eaten at appropriate times of the day, we can avoid the slippery slope of the fast food culture, with its ubiquitous availability, processed carbohydrate, sugar, trans fats and too many calories.

Tip number two: Eat at the table
This is an entirely personal choice but it would help to improve our relationship with food if we could return to eating at the table. There are many benefits to this, such as making mealtimes a more social activity and helping with digestion; similarly, if we can then stop eating between meals and 'grazing', it becomes much easier to keep our calorie intake under control and otherwise avoid overeating. People around the Mediterranean have one of the healthiest diets known to science (with low rates of heart disease and obesity) but appear to eat a lot of food. In fact, they traditionally eat plant-based, real food in relatively small portions at structured family mealtimes around the table. We can learn a lot from these naturally slim, healthy people and eating at the table is a good first step along the way. Even if you are on your own, try to re-connect with more structured eating – set yourself a place, get your favourite book, turn off the computer and the TV for a while and make yourself a proper meal to enjoy at the table. Otherwise, try generally to return to more traditional mealtimes, e.g. Sunday lunch with the

family or a more formal evening meal with your partner. Try and keep the TV dinners to a minimum. ☺

Tip number three: Make sure there is real food in the house
We've all seen the TV weight loss shows where the 'expert' goes into someone's house and berates them about the contents of their food cupboards and fridge. Well, we are going to be a bit more grown up here, so I have listed some groceries and provisions that are helpful to buy before getting underway with the programme. None of this will cost too much and of course, these food staples don't need to be bought in one go. These are mainly the condiments, herbs and spices designed to enhance the flavour and taste of natural, real food meals. Consequently, they will last a long time, which in effect makes them cheap. Here are just some of my suggestions for your store cupboard:

- Extra Virgin Olive oil (ideally from the island of Crete)
- Dijon mustard (the smooth, yellow stuff – for my vinaigrette dressing)
- Various curry spices, e.g. cumin, cardamom, fenugreek, coriander, as well as some commercial curry powder. Try to buy from an Asian grocer (it's cheaper), as and when you need it. Keep spices in sealed jars for freshness.
- White wine vinegar
- Udo's oil (health food shops or online)
- Various seeds, e.g. pumpkin, sunflower and flaxseed (linseed), to sprinkle on salads etc
- Sea salt and black pepper (i.e. pepper cloves in a grinder)

- Organic vegetable stock powder
- Dried (or tinned) organic lentils, chick peas etc
- Rapeseed oil
- Organic brown basmati rice (for an occasional healthy 'treat')
- Tinned fish – tuna, mackerel, sardines etc (try to buy tinned fish in spring water and make sure it is both dolphin-friendly and MSC-approved).
- Quinoa (a true wonder food)
- Some Asian food staples, e.g. rice wine, sesame oil, soy sauce etc

Tip number four: Eat plenty of real food

One of the easiest traps to fall into when trying to lose weight is not eating enough food. Unlike traditional diets, which severely restrict how much we eat, the Back to Basics diet only works if we eat plenty of (mostly plant) food at each meal. We should aim to eventually eat just two meals a day, so make sure to eat plenty of cooked green vegetables and/or salad with your chosen protein to ensure you are full and not going to suffer hunger pangs between meals. Don't worry too much about portion size; this is not a restriction diet. By eating real, natural food and eating until you are comfortably full, the calories will look after themselves. If you do get hungry, have a small real food snack. It is far better to take things slowly and get used to eating a plant-based, real food diet (which will deliver long-term, sustainable weight loss), rather than starving ourselves in the vain hope of a quick fix. That's why traditional diets don't work.

Why this stuff matters

We owe it to ourselves and to those who love us and care about us to improve our health and 'future-proof' ourselves as much as possible. Without going over the science again, there is little doubt that the most effective way to do this is to return to a healthy weight. However, we have been told to 'eat less and move more' or 'cut down' or 'watch our portion size' or 'eat healthily' or 'just take more exercise' ad nauseam for most of our lives. Faced with a barrage of contradictory advice, we have stumbled from one diet to another, taking one step forward and two steps back before eventually losing heart and reverting to our self-imposed misery and another packet of biscuits. I speak from experience!

It's time to put all that in the past. By changing our diet to one comprising real, unprocessed food and starting to take daily activity, our weight will come down and we will start feeling like a much healthier, happier person all round. However, we can do better; by following one of the Back to Basics diet plans, we can maximize our ability to lose weight and ensure that we keep that weight off in the future. Eating plant-based, real, unprocessed foods at set times allows us to reduce our calorie intake and stabilize our insulin levels at a lower level for most of the day. And by taking activity when we are best able to burn fat, we can fit the final piece into the weight loss jigsaw and markedly improve our chances of lifelong, permanent weight loss.

The rules of the game

The Back to Basics programme doesn't rely on fads, weird ingredients or recipes that only a Michelin-starred chef could understand. Nevertheless, to stay on the straight and narrow, it helps to keep a few rules of the game in mind. These 'rules' are just guidelines to help us make the correct choices when shopping, preparing meals at home or eating out, as follows:

- *Stick to real foods* – fruit, salads, vegetables, fish, organic poultry, fresh eggs, nuts, organic meats etc.

- *Avoid all forms of processed foods* – takeaways, sandwiches, ready meals, 'fast foods', breads, cakes, pastries, sugary snacks, savoury snacks, beer, sodas etc.

- *Think before reaching for a sandwich or cake etc* out of habit – stop, breathe, think and act.

- *Eating out is easy* – choose your protein (ideally fish, chicken or vegetarian) and add loads of veggies and salad. Say 'no thank you' to puddings, bread rolls, chips, pints of beer etc. Enjoy your meal, have a glass of wine if you wish and remain safe in the knowledge that you are losing weight and still on your path to health and happiness.

- *Eat loads of green plants* – salads and veggies etc. Eat these foods until you are pleasantly full. If you get hungry between meals, eat more green things.

- *Get active every day* – walk, cycle, swim etc twice a day. Try and get active before eating your first meal of the day and again before your evening meal.

- *Enjoy life* – treasure the good times, love your partner and your kids, see your friends, go out and socialize (follow the rules about eating out!). It's an old cliché but life is not a rehearsal – make the most of every day.

The Back to Basics Modified Programme

A very infirm friend of mine asked me if I could tweak the Back to Basics diet for people like her who, due to injury, illness or disability, are unable to take any activity at all. Here, then, is a slightly modified version of the Basic Programme for those of you who wish to lose weight but are unable to exercise for whatever reason.

What follows is similar to the Basic Programme but with more emphasis on calorie control, an unfortunate necessity, I'm afraid, for those who are unable to exercise. If you wish, you can work out your own BMI (see Appendix 1) and then apply strict calorie counting at each meal. However, that's a complete pain so instead I recommend you follow the Basic Programme but use strict portion control at each meal, e.g. no more food than would fit in one small dessert bowl. Most of us who are obese, regardless of our current ability to be active or not, have got that way through a lifetime's over-consumption of processed foods and sugar. Even if you are unable to take any activity but follow my advice to the letter, you will still be dramatically reducing your calorie consumption compared to the bad old days. Nevertheless, you *will* need to be very careful about portion size and number of snacks. You have very little leeway on your calorie intake if we are to get that weight moving. So, stick to two meals per day and one mid-afternoon snack. Don't worry too much – the wonderful, tasty, natural food you will eat from now on, albeit in fairly concise portions, will still fill you up, reduce your hunger pangs, make you lose weight and above all, make you feel a whole heap better about yourself, too. ☺

Some tips and tricks for the Modified Programme

My advice here is much the same as the Basic Programme. Try to cook like Grandma – buy a good quality joint/chicken, make it last two or three meals, make stock, make soups, grow your own veg etc. Just use any combination of healthy protein, i.e. fish, chicken, turkey, eggs, cheese, or vegetable foods like lentils, chickpeas, hummus etc with lots of salad, veggies etc. Red meat is OK in moderation but there is some evidence that excessive red meat consumption might be carcinogenic, so chicken, fish and vegetable protein is safer. I will allow you some berry fruit for 'afters'. Just concentrate on portion size. We are still just trying to get rid of the sugar (processed carbs) and go back to eating real food. So, if you get really hungry, have another small plant-based snack.

As per the Basic Programme, once you are comfortable with the programme, have a go at creating your own meals to suit you. Keep it simple at first – just combine real, organic protein with lots of salad and/or vegetables. Try having my Wonder Salad at each meal, either as a main course or as a side dish. Make your own version – take it to work, eat it for supper or have it for breakfast. Eat lots of plants!

Here's your plan:

- Alarm clock goes off. Time to face the day.

- Can you do any sort of activity now? This is entirely up to you but there is often something that can be done to raise the heartbeat a bit. When my mother had a hip replacement and couldn't walk for a few weeks, she sat in a chair and did some stretches and arm swinging, all to her favourite music. So, anything you can do now will burn a few calories and make life much easier all round. Don't worry if this is too much – just watch those portion sizes. ☺

- *Breakfast*: Have a cup of tea or coffee if you want but see if you can hold out till later in the morning before eating. I'm not anti-breakfast as such, so if that is simply too difficult, please enjoy a healthy breakfast now.

- *Brunch/Lunch*: Try to make this the first meal of the day. That way, you can maximize your overnight 'fast' before raising your insulin levels again when you eat. If you do eat breakfast, do not eat again until later in the day, i.e. have a late lunch, not a brunch two hours after breakfast. We are just trying to control our calories and let our insulin levels drop back to a resting level as much as possible between meals. Here, though, you have to be very careful about portion size. Remember, one small bowl of food – no more.

- *Afternoon snack*: Try some fresh fruit or raw veggies with hummus or a handful of nuts etc.

- Can you get active again? Sometime in the late afternoon or early evening, try to do some form of activity again, before dinner. Again, this depends entirely on your personal circumstances but have a think about it and see if you can work out some way you can burn a few calories now.

- *Evening meal*: Choose one from – fish with veggies/salad, vegetable protein with veggies/salad, chicken/turkey with veggies/salad etc. (Add spices and flavours as much as you like. Use olive oil or Udo's Oil in moderation for salad dressing and don't worry too much about fat on meat etc). Enjoy a glass of wine if you wish but no pudding – have some fresh fruit instead. Unfortunately, you must be strict with your portions again.

- *Time to relax*: Enjoy some quality time with your partner, family, friends etc. Read a book, watch a movie, talk about your holiday plans and tell your partner how much you love them… It's time to re-discover happiness in life.

- *Bedtime*: Over to you!

Use the same meal/recipe ideas from the Basic Programme but as always, feel free to use your own recipes and meal ideas as you wish. Just stick to the rules of the game and really nail those portion sizes.

Here is a sample two-week plan on the Modified Programme:

Week One	Am activity	Brunch	Snack	Pm activity	Dinner
Monday	Do what you can	Cold chicken, salad/ veggies	Fresh Fruit	Whatever you can	One-Minute Wonder Salad
Tuesday	"	Tuna salad	Nuts and veggies	"	Home-made soup
Wednesday	"	Omelette and salad	Fresh fruit	"	Smoked haddock and veggies
Thursday	"	Vegetable curry	Fresh fruit	"	Quinoa and salad
Friday	"	Salmon salad	Nuts and veggies	"	Dave's daal and veggies
Saturday	"	Bacon and mushrooms	Crudités and hummus	"	Salade Nicoise
Sunday	"	Sunday roast	Fresh fruit	"	Cold cuts and salad

Week Two	Am activity	Brunch	Snack	Pm activity	Dinner
Monday	Do what you can	Turkey and avocado salad	Fresh Fruit	Whatever you can	Easy lamb casserole
Tuesday	"	Greek salad	Nuts and veggies	"	Spicy quinoa
Wednesday	"	Chickpea salad	Fresh fruit	"	Quick spicy beef mince and veggies
Thursday	"	Lentil soup	Fresh fruit	"	Simple Moroccan chicken
Friday	"	Back to Basics Buddha bowl	Nuts and veggies	"	Baked salmon
Saturday	"	Baked curry cauliflower	Crudités and hummus	"	Succulent slow roast lamb
Sunday	"	Tender roast pork	Fresh fruit	"	Cold cuts and salad

The Back to Basics Maintenance Programme

Sticking to the rules of the game

Here is the Maintenance Programme, a guide to follow for life *after* the Back to Basics diet programme(s) or simply a checklist to refer to if and when you want a quick refresher on the specifics of the diet. It takes commitment and no little effort to make the changes achieved so far, so well done for getting to this stage.

If followed carefully over several months, the Basic or Modified Programmes will produce significant weight loss. We don't want to keep losing weight forever though (it costs a fortune in clothes ☺) but neither do we want to undo all the good work by falling back into our bad old ways of disorganized eating and too much processed junk food. What, then, do we need to alter to make the Basic (or Modified) Programme suitable as a lifelong template for weight management and healthy living?

We still need to keep up the daily activity, so the morning activity before brunch/lunch has to stay. In terms of meal planning, I suggest sticking to a late brunch or an early lunch in preference to breakfast. However, if your weight is stable, feel free to have something to eat straight after your morning activity, if you wish. Similarly, the afternoon activity session, before dinner, should also stay. Afternoon snacks are fine as well. What else needs to change? Not much, really. The beauty of the Basic Programme is that it not only helps us lose weight and change our eating habits to be in line with our design as healthy humans, it also serves as our daily guide through life as well. Two meals per day of real, natural, mostly plant-based, unprocessed food plus a fresh fruit or veggie snack, plus daily activity, is all we need to do to remain healthy and happy for the rest of our lives.

The good news is that we can probably relax our portion control a bit and eat more at each meal. Just keep an eye on the weight and if it starts to creep up, go back to 'one dessert bowl' and the extra pounds will soon melt away. Eat plenty of (mostly plant) food and all will be well. From now on, forget about the cakes, pastries, takeaways and junk food that we used to eat in the past. We don't want to stumble now, not after all the progress we have made in recent months. If and when temptation rears its ugly head, a good tip is to take off all your clothes, step on the bedroom scales and have a good look in a full-length mirror. Best to do this in private, probably! For those who still need to lose some weight, this private moment will help focus the mind and keep you motivated in the weeks ahead. For those who have lost loads of weight already and look fantastic and 'beach-ready' in the mirror, it would be criminal to spoil that wonderful feeling by returning to eating cakes and doing no exercise, wouldn't it?

Feel free to experiment and try lots of healthy new recipes but there is no requirement to be a gourmet chef to follow these diet plans. Try my recipes to start with and see how you get on. After that, fill your boots. Just stick to the rules of the game!

12

Final thoughts

I hope you have enjoyed the book and wish you the best of luck with your weight loss journey in future. I have put a lot of emphasis on putting ourselves first in life at various points in the book; this is quite deliberate as our obesity problems stem not only from a bad diet but also from a lack of care and attention to how we eat or otherwise live our lives. Most of us know intuitively that we shouldn't be eating much of the 'food' we eat, even if we don't quite know why. So, let's put ourselves first for a change, certainly in terms of what we eat and when we take activity each day.

We are all unique, wonderful human beings who deserve to be healthy and happy in life. I know the misery that can ensue once we lose control of our eating and drinking and start to pile on the pounds. If nothing else, by taking steps to lose weight and return to full health, our own self-confidence and self-esteem will receive a huge boost. That, all by itself, is a cause for celebration.

The flip side is that it is easy to forget just how many people have our best interests at heart. Even if we are currently at a low ebb, we must not lose sight of the fact that we are loved – probably more than we can imagine. A few years ago, I lost a very dear friend to cancer. She was 57 years old and rather famous in her own right. At her funeral, mourners stood ten deep outside the crematorium; five hundred people attended her memorial service. Her husband, so obviously devastated himself, remarked that she would never have believed how many people came to see her off. That was because many, many people loved her, far more than she would have ever realized when she was alive. And that goes for us too. Although getting our diet and lifestyle right is important, there is more to life than food. We should take the time to re-connect with the important people in our lives, spend time with them, laugh with them and share meals and wine together (real food meals only, please!) and remember that life is for living. Let's cherish each and every day we are alive and not feel guilty about taking these steps to lose weight and boost our health. All we are really doing is ensuring that people who love us have us around for as long as possible. And vice versa, of course. ☺

Many thanks for reading the book.

13

Recipes

I have listed some of my favourite recipes here (including the relevant recipes for the two-week diet plan templates), grouped under the headings of 'Super quick and easy brunches' and 'Quick and easy dinners'. This is not a rigid list but a basic guide to help with meal planning in the early stages. Please experiment with other recipes and food combinations as you go along; this is a template for life, so it helps to embrace as many different recipes and ways to combine real food as much as possible in the months and years ahead. The recipes described below are mainly designed for two people, with the exception of the more family-orientated meals, such as the roast pork etc. Here are just a few suggestions to get the ball rolling:

Super quick and easy brunches
- Astronaut's breakfast
- Mushroom omelette
- Scrambled eggs and bacon
- Scrambled eggs and smoked salmon
- Smoked haddock and poached egg
- Kedgeree
- 'One-Minute Wonder Salad' (recipe in 'Dinners' section)

- Turkey and avocado salad
- Mackerel salad
- Chickpea salad
- Lentil soup
- Baked curry cauliflower
- Lentil salad
- Back to Basics Buddha bowl

Quick and easy dinners

- Roast chicken
- Healthy chicken and veggie soup
- Veggie curry
- 'One-Minute Wonder Salad'
- Gilly's wonderful Asian fish
- Quinoa salad
- Tarka daal
- Salade Nicoise
- My vinaigrette
- Asian broccoli
- Tender roastpork
- Quick spicy beef mince
- Easy lamb casserole
- Simple Moroccan chicken
- Baked salmon
- Greek salad
- Succulent slow roast lamb
- Spicy quinoa
- Home-made gravy
- Home-made mint sauce

Super quick and easy brunches

Astronaut's breakfast

This is the breakfast eaten by the NASA astronauts in the Apollo era. It is ideal for a special weekend treat.

Ingredients
- An organic beef steak (fillet or sirloin)
- A knob of organic butter
- Salt and pepper
- One or two fresh organic eggs
- Some organic butter
- Rapeseed oil
- White wine vinegar

Take a small organic piece of beef fillet steak or sirloin steak and season with salt and pepper. Heat a teaspoon of oil in a frying pan and turn up the heat. Add a knob of organic butter. When it has stopped foaming, place the steak in the pan. Cook a couple of minutes each side or otherwise to taste. Meanwhile, boil some water in a saucepan. Add a teaspoon of white wine vinegar and a little salt and crack one or two eggs in to the pan. Immediately remove from the heat and cover. When the steak is cooked, let it rest on a warm plate until the eggs are poached (about three minutes). Eat at the table and imagine you are about to walk on the moon.

Mushroom Omelette

Ingredients
- Three fresh organic eggs
- Some sliced organic mushrooms
- Some organic butter
- Sea salt and pepper and some dried mixed herbs

Break three organic eggs into a bowl and beat gently with a fork. Season with salt and pepper and add a pinch of dried herbs. Melt a little organic butter in a small frying pan and gently sauté some sliced, organic mushrooms until they are soft. Pour in the eggs and when they start to set, tip the pan forward and push the eggs into the middle of the pan with a spatula. Tip the pan backwards a little and pull the egg mixture to middle of pan again. When the eggs are just about to set, fold over the omelette and tip onto a warm plate. Have a portion of Wonder Salad on the side for a delicious, healthy brunch or supper.

Scrambled eggs (with bacon or smoked salmon)

Very popular in our house, I make these all the time. I think I got the idea from Elizabeth David many years ago but I suspect this is another generic recipe.

Ingredients
- Two or three very fresh organic eggs.
- A knob of organic butter
- Salt and white pepper

- A good quality saucepan
- A clear kitchen mixing bowl
- Wooden spoon

Crack the eggs into the mixing bowl, season with salt and white pepper and beat quickly with a fork. Melt butter in saucepan on a low heat. When butter is starting to foam, tip in the eggs and stir continuously with the wooden spoon. Now comes the tricky bit – eggs cook quickly and continue to cook when the pan is removed from the heat, so you have to anticipate a bit here. When the eggs just start to 'scramble' but before you think they are ready, remove the pan from the heat. Keep stirring. Add another small knob of butter and another twist of white pepper. One more stir and you are done. Eat the eggs on their own or with some bacon perhaps (you can cook bacon in about two minutes in a microwave) or some beautiful sliced organic smoked salmon for a special treat.

Smoked haddock

Ingredients
- A nice fillet of smoked haddock (the natural smoked fish – not the artificial bright yellow variety)
- Some skimmed milk
- A knob of organic butter
- Salt and pepper

Place the fish in a saucepan and cover with the milk. Add the butter and a twist of salt and pepper. Cover and cook gently for about ten minutes (if the heat is too high, the milk will boil over). Serve with loads of steamed veggies or have with a couple of poached eggs as a delicious brunch dish.

Kedgeree

I try to steer clear of rice, as (white) rice is a processed carb with a high GI rating (quinoa is a great rice substitute). However, this dish makes a delicious weekend brunch and by using unprocessed brown rice, we keep the GI down anyway. This is my quick version of a classic recipe.

Ingredients
- A small piece of smoked haddock
- Two organic, free-range eggs
- One medium onion, finely chopped
- About half a litre of hot organic vegetable stock (made from stock powder)
- 1 teaspoon of mild curry powder and ½ teaspoon of turmeric
- Half a pint of skimmed milk
- Fresh parsley
- Organic butter
- Most of a small packet of organic brown basmati rice (about 300–400grams)
- Fresh lemon and salt and pepper

Cook the smoked haddock as per my earlier recipe. Boil the eggs in a saucepan of water until just hard-boiled (about eight minutes). Cook the onion in some butter until softened. Stir in the turmeric and curry powder and cook for one minute. Add the rice and stir thoroughly to coat each grain with the mixture. Add the stock and stir gently. Bring to the boil then turn heat right down, cover and leave for about ten minutes. Check occasionally – just cook until the rice is tender and all the liquid has been absorbed. Add more stock if necessary.

When the rice is cooked, remove skin (and any bones) from the smoked haddock and flake into bite-sized pieces with a fork. Peel the eggs and chop into small pieces as well. Stir fish and eggs into the rice mixture and gently fold in. Warm through on the hob for a couple of minutes. Add some chopped parsley, a twist of salt and pepper and you're done. Serve with a small side salad. Delicious!

Turkey and avocado salad

Ingredients
- 3 large slices of turkey (most supermarket deli counters will slice this fresh for you)
- ½ a ripe avocado
- Super side salad (spinach, rocket, lettuce, tomato, watercress, cucumber, olives)

Slice the avocado into thick wedges and place on a small dinner plate with the turkey. Make my vinaigrette in a salad bowl and toss the other salad ingredients together (ideally fresh or just supermarket bags of salad ingredients). Pile loads of salad on the plate (try to fill about 80% of the plate with salad) and you are done. I always have a little English mustard on the side but that's just my taste. This makes a simple brunch or supper dish and is ideal to take to work in a suitable container, too.

Mackerel salad

You can use smoked or tinned mackerel for this recipe, whichever you prefer. Grilled fresh mackerel is best of all but sometimes hard to source.

Ingredients
- A piece of smoked mackerel or tin of mackerel
- 1 large slice of rye bread (folded over for sandwich)
- Portion of Wonder Salad
- Vinaigrette

Assemble on a plate, dress salad with vinaigrette. Or make a sandwich with rye bread, mackerel and salad filling. Ideal to take to work.

Chickpea salad

Ingredients
- ½ a tin of pre-cooked chickpeas
- A handful of cherry tomatoes
- A bag of washed baby spinach
- Some rocket
- ½ clove garlic
- Vinaigrette dressing

Rub the garlic gently and quickly around the inside of a salad bowl or other salad container (you just want a hint of garlic – do not overpower the dish). Make a bed of spinach in the bowl, add the rocket and cherry tomatoes and dress with the vinaigrette. Put the chickpeas on top, season with a twist of sea salt and ground black pepper and you are ready to go. Again, ideal in a container for work. Have with one slice of rye bread on the side if you wish.

Lentil soup

Ingredients
- One onion, finely chopped
- Clove garlic, finely chopped
- A stick of celery, chopped
- One teaspoon of mild curry powder
- ½ teaspoon smoked paprika
- 250 grams red lentils, washed
- 400g tin of chopped tomatoes (ideally organic)
- Olive oil
- One litre vegan stock
- Salt and pepper

This is a very easy soup to make and a fantastic and filling soup for a winter's day. You can make this ahead of time, keep in the fridge and just warm up whatever quantity you need. Take in a soup flask to work if appropriate.

Wash the lentils in a bowl under a slow running cold tap until water runs clean. Drain and reserve. Make up one litre of vegan stock with boiling water (vegan stock powder is sold in health food shops and many supermarkets these days). Sauté onion and garlic in a little olive oil in a large saucepan over a medium heat for about five minutes or until onions are soft and translucent. Add the celery and cook for another two minutes. Add the curry powder and paprika and cook through for one minute.

Add the stock to the saucepan, along with the lentils and tin of tomatoes. Bring to the boil and skim off any scum that comes to the surface. Turn down the heat, put the lid on and simmer for about 45 minutes. Season to taste and enjoy.

Baked curry cauliflower

Ingredients
- 200 ml Vegan stock
- One cauliflower, chopped into florets
- One red onion
- Tsp mild curry powder
- Tsp Cumin seeds
- ½ tsp Garam masala
- ½ tsp turmeric
- ½ green chili – chopped and seeds removed (optional)
- Fresh coriander
- A little grapeseed oil
- Salt and pepper

There are lots of famous curries which feature cauliflower in some way or another (Aloo Gobi is probably the most famous). This is my quick and easy 'curried cauliflower' brunch dish, inspired by all those ghee-filled curries we love so much.

Preheat oven to 200ºC or 180ºC in a fan oven. Put pan of water on to boil and blanch cauliflower in the boiling water for about two minutes. Drain in colander and reserve.

Chop red onion into rings and sauté in a little oil in a frying pan until caramelized. This will take about twenty minutes. Watch onions carefully – it is easy to go over and make them bitter. Spread cauliflower in single layer on a baking tray (use a non-stick baking tray liner ideally). Pour over enough stock to soak cauliflower and leave a little extra on the liner. Add the caramelized onion and then dust cauliflower with the curry powder, cumin, turmeric and garam masala. Add a twist of black pepper and some sea salt. Add a few slices of green chilli if using (can be quite hot so up to you). Mix the cauliflower with the spices using a wooden spoon to make sure each floret is well covered in the spice mix. Mix should be quite wet at this point. Add more stock if necessary.

Bake in oven until tender (between 20 and 30 minutes but check regularly with a sharp knife). Top up with stock during cooking if necessary. Don't overcook or the cauliflower will turn to mush.

When cooked, sprinkle chopped fresh coriander over the cauliflower and serve with side salad and/or some steamed veggies. Have a spoonful of brown rice if you wish.

Lentil salad

This is a very quick brunch dish that includes one of the only form of processed foods I approve of, i.e. pre-packed lentils.

Ingredients
- ½ onion, finely chopped
- ½ clove garlic
- Olive oil
- Salad ingredients of your choice (e.g. tomatoes, spinach, lettuce, chopped celery, cucumber) or some steamed kale
- Packet of pre-cooked Puy lentils (the dark, earthy ones)
- A sprig of thyme
- Some vegan stock (about 200 ml)

Quick version: make up a salad in a bowl with your chosen salad ingredients and dress with a vinaigrette or other dressing of your choice. If you prefer, steam some kale in a saucepan with a little boiling water and have that instead of or as well as the salad. Zap the packet of lentils in the microwave and leave to cool. Mix the lentils with the salad ingredients in a large bowl and season to taste.

More sophisticated version: make up salad (and/or steamed kale) as above. Fry onion and garlic until soft in a little olive oil in saucepan over a medium heat. Zap lentils in microwave for about thirty seconds, let cool a little then open packet and add lentils to the saucepan with the stock and sprig of thyme.

Simmer for about ten minutes. Drain lentils and cool for about twenty minutes. Season to taste. Mix lentils with salad as before or layer on top of steamed kale. One slice of rye bread makes a good accompaniment.

Back to Basics Buddha bowl

I know that Buddha bowls are all the rage these days and I have certainly become a big fan of this way of eating in recent years. It is a clever way to combine mainly plant foods in an attractive and tasty fashion, whilst using the bowl to control portion size. There are numerous Buddha bowl recipes out there but here is just one example to try:

Ingredients
- One dessert bowl
- Baby spinach
- Rocket
- Chopped cos lettuce
- One avocado, flesh scooped out and sliced
- Some quinoa cooked in vegan stock
- Hummus
- Your choice of topping, e.g. cooked chicken, tuna, baked chickpeas, baked sweet potato, roasted carrots

Assemble Buddha bowl as follows:
Make a 'nest' in the bottom of the bowl with the spinach, rocket and lettuce. Try to fill half the bowl with the salad ingredients.

Add some cooked quinoa, a spoonful of hummus and the sliced avocado. Top off with veggie or protein of your choice.

P.S. You can roast a potato/sweet potatoes/chickpeas etc in the oven in a variety of spices to taste. I often cover a tray of chickpeas in curry powder, a little olive oil and a small amount of chopped garlic plus salt and pepper and bake in oven on a high heat for about ten minutes. This makes a great bowl topping.

Quick and easy dinners

Roast chicken

Ingredients
- One or two fresh organic chickens
- Some organic butter
- An onion, peeled and cut in half
- A selection of vegetables, e.g. carrots, cabbage, broccoli, cauliflower
- Salt and pepper

Take the chicken out of the fridge in good time (it needs to be at room temperature) and wash it inside and out under the tap. Put a bit of organic butter inside the cavity with the two onion halves and sprinkle a bit of sea salt and pepper over the skin. Roast at about 190°C for 20 minutes to the pound plus twenty minutes. Baste regularly and you will end up with a perfect roast chicken. Steam the veggies (I just put half an inch of water in the bottom of a saucepan but you can buy a proper steamer if you wish) to preserve all the vitamins and phytonutrients. Add a portion Wonder salad and you have a delicious, healthy Sunday lunch for up to four people for less than the cost of eating out at a fast food restaurant.

Healthy chicken and veggie soup

Ingredients
- Some earthy vegetables, e.g. carrot, onion, celery, leek, small potato
- Some fresh herbs (to your taste)
- An onion, peeled and cut in half.
- A bay leaf
- Some organic butter
- Salt and pepper
- A handful of red lentils
- Chicken carcass

Start by making a stock, so fill a big saucepan with cold water and place the chicken carcass in the pan. Add a carrot, an onion cut in two, a piece of celery and maybe a leek etc. Add a little salt and pepper. You could try a few herbs in the stock as well? Bring to the boil, remove any scum that forms with a slotted spoon and then simmer for about two hours (put the lid on). Let the stock cool and then strain into a bowl or jug through a sieve (sounds complicated but it really isn't and if you do this when you first get home, it will be ready in time for dinner). Chop up some more veggies (ideally, celery, onions, carrots, maybe a small potato) and sweat in a little butter in a saucepan for about twenty minutes. Add a little sea salt and black pepper then pour in the stock. Add a handful of red lentils and a few shreds of leftover chicken and simmer for twenty minutes. Eat as is or liquidize, as you wish.

Veggie curry

There is any number of recipes for a good curry but this is my super quick version. You can make it in ten minutes, with a bit of practice.

Ingredients
- Two or three onions
- Tin of organic chickpeas
- Assorted vegetables, e.g. celery, carrot, peas, runner beans, cauliflower
- Cumin seeds
- Cardamom pods
- A clove of garlic, finely chopped
- A piece of fresh ginger, finely chopped
- A teaspoon of commercial curry powder
- Rapeseed oil
- Organic vegetable stock powder
- Organic brown basmati rice, cooked as per instructions on the packet

Roughly chop up two or three onions, pop them in a saucepan, cover with boiling water from the kettle and bring to the boil. Turn the heat down and simmer for about seven minutes. Meanwhile, open a tin of organic chickpeas, chop up the veggies and put the whole lot in another saucepan, cover with boiling water and simmer until just soft (about five minutes). Drain when cooked. While the onions/ veggies are cooking, grind up the cumin seeds, cardamom pod, garlic, fresh ginger and curry powder (which can be 'mild, 'medium', 'hot', 'Madras' etc, entirely up to you) in a pestle and mortar. When the onions are cooked, drain them and puree in a bowl with a hand-held blender. Put a little rapeseed oil in the original pan and return to the heat – add the pureed onions and tip in the ground up spice mixture from the pestle and mortar. Give the pan a stir and then mix up about a third of a pint of organic vegetable stock powder with boiling water from the kettle. Stir the drained veggies into the onion/spice pan. Add the vegetable stock. Cook for a further two minutes, check for seasoning and you are done. Have with a portion of organic brown basmati rice (the type you cook in a packet in a microwave will do, if necessary) and a large salad.

One-Minute Wonder Salad

This is my go-to dish that often forms the basis of many meals. It is great as a large standalone portion for lunch or supper or as a smaller portion as a side dish with dinner. It is easy to take to work in a plastic food box, too – just add a tin of tuna, some hard-boiled eggs or a piece of cold chicken for the perfect lunch, supper or office meal. I use a salad spinner to wash and dry the lettuce; they are a great investment (try Lakeland for such things – www.lakeland.co.uk). This salad can be made in just one minute, provided everything is to hand in the kitchen.

Ingredients
- Three tsp organic extra virgin olive oil (from Crete)
- One tsp white wine vinegar
- One tsp Dijon mustard (the smooth yellow variety – not the grainy one)
- Half tsp of sea salt and twist of black pepper
- One cos (or Romaine) lettuce
- Tomatoes
- Cucumber
- A red onion
- A packet of baby spinach
- Some rocket
- Fresh coriander
- Any pre-cooked veggies, e.g. cauliflower florets, broccoli
- A tin of organic chickpeas

In a salad bowl, mix three teaspoons of Cretan extra virgin olive oil with one teaspoon of lemon juice or white wine vinegar. Stir in half a teaspoon of Dijon mustard (the smooth yellow stuff, not the grainy one). Add a twist of black pepper. Chop up a cos lettuce and chuck into your salad spinner. Rinse under the tap and spin vigorously. Tip the chopped-up lettuce into the salad bowl. Grab a kitchen knife and a chopping board (watch your fingers). Chop the following quickly and add to the salad bowl – some fresh tomatoes, half a cucumber, a red onion, some baby spinach (packet?), some rocket (packet?), some fresh coriander, any spare veggies, e.g. some pre-cooked broccoli florets, cauliflower. Open a tin of organic chickpeas, drain and tip some into the bowl (keep the rest for the curry). Mix thoroughly with wooden salad spoons and that's it.

Gilly's wonderful Asian fish

My sister Gilly has long been cajoling me to eat more fish. She is the perfect example of why we should all eat fish on a regular basis – slim, fit, in perfect health and looking about twenty years younger than her true age. I'm not sure where she got this recipe (it is probably fairly generic) but it is easy and quick to make and absolutely delicious. Try to source really fresh fish for this recipe -see my list of recommended suppliers in the Appendix. Serve with loads of steamed vegetables.

Ingredients
- Fresh fillet of white fish (e.g. plaice, sole, sea bass etc)
- Two spring onions, finely chopped
- One clove of garlic, finely chopped
- Some fresh ginger, finely chopped
- One red chilli, finely chopped
- Dash of rice wine
- Dash of soy sauce
- Dash of sesame oil

- Twist of black pepper
- A sheet of cooking 'foil'

Wash the fish and place in the centre of the foil. Cover with all the other ingredients. Fold the foil over the fish and scrunch up to make a sealed parcel. Place in fridge and leave to marinate overnight. When ready to cook, pre-heat oven to about 170ºC. Place foil parcel on baking tray and cook for twenty minutes. Be careful when opening the parcel – don't scald yourself. Serve with steamed veggies.

Quinoa salad

I absolutely love quinoa and eat it about three times a week. It is one of the most nutritious of all vegetarian foods and is really versatile in terms of cooking and incorporating into other dishes. A very simple way to eat quinoa is to cook a portion and have it as a side dish, in lieu of potatoes or rice, for instance. Anyway, here is a super quick quinoa recipe, as follows.

Ingredients
- A cup of organic quinoa (most supermarkets stock this nowadays)
- A teaspoon of organic vegetable stock powder
- One medium onion, finely chopped
- Some organic butter
- About half a pint of boiling water from the kettle
- One saucepan

Melt some butter in the saucepan over a low heat and sauté the onion until soft. Tip the quinoa into the saucepan. Add about half a pint of boiling water from the kettle. Stir in a teaspoon of organic vegetable stock powder. Cover and cook gently until all the water is absorbed (about five minutes). Remove the lid and dry out the quinoa for a minute or so on a low heat. Fluff up with a fork and serve in a bowl. Try with Asian broccoli or a large Wonder Salad.

Tarka daal

I found this recipe on the internet years ago but I can't remember whose it was originally. If you're reading, please accept my apologies but as it is such a good recipe, I would like your permission to repeat it here.

Ingredients
- 9oz red lentils
- 1.5 teaspoons ground cumin
- 0.5 teaspoon turmeric
- I teaspoon grated ginger (try 'Very Lazy Ginger' in a jar from the supermarket)
- I red onion
- Lots of chopped fresh coriander
- 3 cloves garlic (finely chopped)
- Cumin seeds
- Rapeseed Oil
- A suitable pan (a famous French cast iron elliptical pan is best)

Wash the lentils, then place in a pan on the hob with the ground cumin, grated ginger and 35fl oz boiling water. Bring to the boil then cook, uncovered, for 20 minutes. You will get a lot of yellow scum on the top – just scoop it off with a spoon. Then, turn heat down to the lowest setting, put the lid on and leave for 3 hours.

Near the end of the cooking time, slice the red onion into very thin rounds and fry in a frying pan in the sunflower oil until caramelized. This is the crucial step for a perfect daal – the onions should be almost burnt and give off a toffee-sort of flavor. Use a slotted spoon to collect the onions (to drain the oil) and put into the lentil mixture. I add quite a large shot of salt, followed by the chopped coriander.

To finish, heat more oil in the same frying pan you used for the onions and sauté the garlic. As it starts to brown, bung in a goodly amount of cumin seeds- fry for a minute and then pour the whole mixture into the daal. Give it a very quick stir and then put the lid back on immediately to seal in the flavour. Serve hot with steamed vegetables and/or a small portion of organic brown basmati rice.

Salade Nicoise

A great classic French dish, suitable for either brunch or dinner. Enjoy with a glass of chilled rosé on a summers day with friends and family and it will feel like being in the South of France!

Ingredients
- One tin of tuna (in olive oil)

- A small tin of anchovies
- Two fresh organic eggs
- Two tomatoes
- A lettuce, washed
- A handful of green beans ('haricot verts')
- A red onion, sliced into rings
- Some black olives
- Fresh basil

In no particular order: Cook the eggs until hard-boiled in a separate pan of water. Top and tail the beans and blanch them in a pan of salted, boiling water for only a minute. Drain and set aside. Mix up one serving of my vinaigrette in the bottom of a steep-sided salad bowl. Chop the lettuce and tomatoes and mix in the salad bowl with the olives and sliced red onion until fully coated with vinaigrette. Arrange the salad mixture on a large plate. Quickly sauté the blanched beans in a saucepan with a tablespoon of water and a knob of butter (for no more than one minute), drain and add to the salad. Shell the eggs, cut into halves and place on the salad. Drain the tuna and place in the middle of the salad. Drain the anchovies and drape around the salad, here and there. Finally, sprinkle with chopped basil and pour over a little more vinaigrette over the whole salad. Voila!

My vinaigrette

This vinaigrette is a vital addition to many salads, including my Salade Nicoise.

Ingredients
- Three tsp organic Cretan extra virgin olive oil
- One tsp white wine vinegar
- One tsp Dijon mustard (the smooth yellow variety – not the grainy one)
- Half tsp sea salt and twist of black pepper

Mix all the ingredients together in the bottom of a deep wooden salad bowl. I use the back of a spoon to mix the mustard through thoroughly. Mix in a bowl and keep in a sealed jar in the fridge if you want but I just make it fresh each time I need it.

Asian broccoli

Use tenderstem broccoli and steam until just tender over a pan of boiling water. In another pan, gently sauté some sliced garlic in olive oil – don't get the oil too hot or it will become unpleasant. When the broccoli is just cooked, drain and then tip into the pan with the garlic and toss on a high heat for a minute or so. Add a dash of good quality soy sauce and serve immediately.

Tender roast pork

This is a traditional lunch for all the family on a Sunday or other special occasion. I think it better generally to replace red meat with other sources of protein (e.g. fish, poultry and vegetable proteins) but my wife loves this dish, so I make it quite often to keep her happy. ☺

The secret to the perfect roast is to start with the best

possible ingredients. That means making friends with your butcher or farm shop and getting hold of the best quality cut of meat you can. For this dish, my preference is for loin of pork on the bone, although belly of pork is also very tasty. Although this is not a cheap meal, the leftovers can be used to make at least one, if not two days' worth of tasty meals to follow, so it is actually a very economical way to eat.

Ingredients
- One joint of free-range loin of pork on the bone (try to source a rare breed such as Gloucester Old Spot)
- Some sea salt
- A handful of sage
- A large array of vegetables of your choice, e.g. cauliflower, carrots, broccoli, Savoy cabbage
- Homemade pork stock or a good quality pork stock cube
- A hairdryer (!)

Take the joint out of the fridge in good time and turn the oven up to max. Whilst the oven is heating up, plug your chosen hairdryer into a suitable socket in the kitchen. (I find it best, if one is going to borrow said hairdryer from one's partner, to ask permission first ☺; similarly, any muck is best wiped off the hairdryer prior to its return – tends to make for a more pleasant ambience at dinner!) Place joint in a suitable oven-proof roasting tin (the heavy cast iron French ones are best) and turn the hairdryer up to full chat. Play the hot air over the skin for a few minutes, until it is absolutely bone dry (ask your butcher to score the skin and 'chine' the joint when you buy).

Once the oven is up to temperature, rub some crushed sea salt over the dried skin of the joint, sprinkle a few sage leaves into the roasting dish and place in the oven. Give it twenty minutes on max, then turn the heat down to about 190ºC (170ºC in a fan oven) and cook for 30 minutes per pound. About twenty minutes from cooked, steam your choice of veggies in a suitable steamer. When the pork is ready, take it out of the oven with oven gloves and transfer to a carving dish. Drain off most of the fat from the roasting tin and then place the roasting tin over a medium heat on the hob. Stir in some stock and some of the vegetable water (a slug of red wine is good, too) and reduce to a 'jus'. Let the pork rest for a few minutes, then carve it up and serve with large chunks of perfect crackling. Enjoy with loads of veggies and some jus. I don't eat it myself but apple sauce is a popular accompaniment with this as well.

Quick spicy beef mince

For those who must get a meat fix now and again, this is a tasty and very quick dinner to prepare, with a side of vegetables and avocado.

Ingredients
- ½ onion, finely chopped
- ½ kg lean beef mince
- 1 tsp olive oil
- 1 tsp cumin powder
- ½ tsp garlic salt
- 1 tsp Creole seasoning

- 200 ml hot beef stock (made from real stock or good quality stock cube)

Sauté the onion in olive oil over a medium heat until soft. Turn up the heat and add the beef mince. Fry for about ten minutes or until the beef is cooked through. Stir regularly. Add the spices and stir through; cook for one minute. Add the hot stock and reduce heat. Simmer for another ten minutes and check the seasoning (it might just need a twist of pepper). Serve with steamed broccoli and ½ avocado, flesh scooped out and sliced. I recommend an accompaniment of one glass Cabernet Sauvignon. ☺

Easy lamb casserole

You can make this at the weekend and then keep a portion in the fridge for use on Monday evening, perhaps.

Ingredients
- 1 onion, chopped
- 600 g lamb loin or shoulder, cut into bite-sized pieces and fat trimmed or removed.
- Olive oil
- 400 g tin organic chopped tomatoes
- 1 celery stick, chopped
- 1 litre hot lamb stock
- 1 small glass red or dry white wine
- Small sprig fresh rosemary
- Salt and pepper

Preheat oven to 190°C. Season the lamb pieces with salt and pepper (most recipes include white flour at this point but I try to avoid this if I can). Heat the olive oil in a large good-quality non-stick pan. Gently fry the lamb pieces (in batches) until browned all over. Transfer the lamb to a casserole dish. Add a touch more olive oil and fry the onion in the pan until nearly caramelized. Transfer onions to the casserole dish. Deglaze frying pan with the wine and pour into the casserole. Add the celery, tomatoes, hot stock and rosemary to the casserole, then cover and place in preheated oven for about one to one and a half hours (a slow cooker makes this easier and results in beautifully moist and tender lamb).

When cooked, check seasoning and adjust with salt and pepper as required. Serve with lots of steamed veggies.

Simple Moroccan chicken

There are more elaborate versions of this dish but this is my quick and easy version, suitable for a weekday night or when time is of the essence.

Ingredients
- 1 onion, finely chopped
- 1 clove garlic, finely chopped
- 2 chicken breasts (ideally organic or at least free-range), skin removed
- ½ inch piece of fresh ginger, peeled and finely chopped (you can buy similar in glass jars from most supermarkets)
- 1 tsp paprika

- 1 tsp ground cumin
- ½ tsp turmeric
- 1 tsp cinnamon
- 1 glass white wine
- A handful of raisins (optional)
- A few green olives, pitted (optional)
- 500 ml hot chicken stock
- A little olive oil
- Bunch of fresh coriander, chopped
- Salt and freshly ground black pepper

Mix all the spices (minus the ginger) on a plate and coat the chicken pieces in the spice mixture. Leave to rest while you get on with the rest of the dish.

Gently heat a little olive oil in a large non-stick saucepan. Fry onion and garlic until just soft. Add ginger and continue to cook for another two minutes. Turn up the heat and add chicken pieces. Cook until browned all over (about ten minutes). Add white wine and cook until alcohol has evaporated. Add the hot stock plus olives and raisins (if using). Turn heat down and simmer gently for about 40 minutes.

Check chicken is cooked through (I use a digital temperature probe). Add chopped coriander to chicken dish and check seasoning. Serve with veggies of choice and some spicy quinoa.

Baked salmon

Ingredients
- 2 fresh salmon steaks

- 1 tbsp honey (runny version)
- 1 tsp Dijon mustard
- 1 tsp balsamic vinegar
- A squeeze of fresh lemon
- Salt and pepper

Preheat oven to 170°C. Mix honey, mustard and lemon juice in a small bowl. Pour over salmon steaks. Season to taste. Place on a lined baking tray and cook in oven for about 20 minutes or until fish flakes easily. Serve with salad, steamed veggies and/or a small portion of brown rice.

Greek salad

Ingredients
- One Romaine lettuce, washed and chopped
- 2 tomatoes, quartered.
- Small red onion, finely sliced
- Green pepper, de-seeded and sliced
- ½ cucumber, chopped into small pieces
- A few pitted olives
- A large chunk of feta cheese
- Best quality organic virgin olive oil
- ½ fresh lemon
- Twist of pepper
- Dried oregano

Assemble all the salad ingredients plus onion on a large dinner plate. Place feta on top. Squeeze lemon over salad and then drizzle olive oil over the cheese and onto the salad (or dress salad with a vinaigrette – your choice). Add a twist of pepper and sprinkle dried oregano on top of cheese.

Succulent slow roast lamb

I like lamb as it is very tasty and common here where I live, up in the hills. The animals have a good free-range life, too.

Ingredients
- One whole or half shoulder of lamb (ideally sourced locally and in season and not from the other side of the world!)
- Fresh rosemary
- Some olive oil
- Salt and pepper
- Homemade gravy: hot lamb stock, a glass of red wine, gravy browning (see below)
- Homemade mint sauce: fresh mint, white wine vinegar, salt and a little sugar or honey (see below)
- Lots of veggies of your choice (e.g. cabbage, broccoli, green beans, cauliflower, carrots

Preheat oven to 200ºC.

Weigh lamb joint then rub with olive oil and season with salt and pepper. Place in a suitable roasting pan. Pierce skin with a sharp knife in several places. Put small sprigs of rosemary in the cut skin and around the joint in the roasting tin.

Place in preheated oven for twenty minutes. Turn heat down to 160°C. Cover joint with foil and cook for at least another two hours. Cook for not less than ½ hour per pound plus twenty minutes, which for a whole shoulder will probably be nearer three hours to be best. Remove from oven, transfer to a dinner plate or serving platter and let rest for about an hour somewhere warm.

The meat should pull away from the bone, so serve in chunks with lots of steamed veggies, some hot homemade gravy and the mint sauce.

Home made gravy

My wife is from the north of England, where gravy isn't right unless it holds a fork upright in the jug but I'm from London originally, so this is my soft southern healthy version, with no added flour.

While the joint is resting, pour off the fat from the roasting tin, leaving just the meat juice behind. Place pan over medium heat on the hob and deglaze pan with wine. Add about ½ litre of lamb stock and bring to the simmer. Add a dash of gravy browning if you wish. Reduce until an appropriate consistency (anywhere between a 'jus' and a London 'gravy', depending on preference).

Watch the seasoning – ideally, try to use real lamb stock, either homemade or from the butcher or supermarket as stock cubes can be very salty. Real stock is fine; just season to taste.

Homemade mint sauce

Ingredients
- A large bunch of fresh mint leaves
- A dash of white wine vinegar
- A tsp of cold water
- A pinch of salt
- Either a few grains of sugar (sugar?? Well, it is Sunday, after all) OR ½ tsp of honey

Chop mint leaves very finely with a cook's knife on a chopping board. Place in small ramekin dish with the vinegar, a little cold water, the salt and sugar grains or honey. Let steep for about an hour before serving.

Spicy quinoa

Ingredients
- A little olive oil
- ½ clove garlic, finely chopped
- ½ red onion, finely chopped
- One tomato, cut into small pieces
- ½ green chilli, seeds removed and finely chopped (optional)
- ½ tsp ground cumin
- One spring onion, finely chopped
- 150 g uncooked quinoa (washed and drained)
- A few red chilli flakes (optional)
- Fresh coriander, roughly chopped

- 500 ml vegan stock

Preheat oven to lowest setting. Wash quinoa in a sieve or colander under a running cold tap for thirty seconds and allow to drain. Heat oil in a large saucepan and gently sauté the onion and garlic until soft. Add the quinoa, cumin, green chilli (if using) and the stock. Adjust amount of stock until the liquid is about 1.5 cm above level of the quinoa. Stir once. Bring to the boil, then turn heat right down, cover and simmer very gently until all liquid is absorbed. Test quinoa now – it should be cooked through and soft. If still a bit hard, add a little more stock and continue cooking. When cooked, place saucepan in the oven to steam out and dry (about an hour ideally).

Let quinoa cool until just warm. Spoon into a warm serving dish and separate grains with a fork. Fold in the spring onion, tomato and fresh coriander. Sprinkle a few red chilli flakes over the quinoa, if you wish. Serve with a large portion of Wonder Salad.

Appendix 1

Basal Metabolic Rate (BMR)

One way we can clear up a common misunderstanding about our calorie requirements is to look at something called the Basal Metabolic Rate or BMR. Your BMR is a measure of the number of calories you need to keep you alive in any 24-hour day, before you do any exercise; in other words, the energy your body needs to keep functioning healthily. If you stayed in bed all day (alone!), you would pretty much burn up the calories as determined by your own BMR plus a bit, which varies in line with your age, your sex, your weight, your height etc. Unfortunately, calculating your own BMR involves a rather scary sum! You don't have to do this but it makes sense to establish your own BMR before going any further. How do we calculate our BMR? Grab a calculator and take a deep breath (see page 212).

You can work out your own BMR if you wish, to help you calculate an appropriate daily calorie intake. However, if you follow the advice and tips of the Back to Basics plan closely, you will reduce your calorie consumption anyway. If you then take plenty of daily activity, you will easily expend more calories than you burn through exercise. With a bit of practice, you will soon find your own balance as to how much food to eat (versus daily activity) to guarantee permanent weight loss.

BASAL METABOLIC RATE
(Equations courtesy of www.bmi-calculator.net):

For a woman, do this sum:
- 655 + (4.35 × your weight in pounds) + (4.7 × your height in inches) – (4.7 × your age in years) = BMR

For a man:
- 66 + (6.23 × your weight in pounds) + (12.7 × your height in inches) – (6.8 × your age in years) = BMR

As an example, imagine a 40-year-old female who is 65 inches tall and weighs 200 pounds (14.3 stones). Crunching the numbers, the equation gives us a BMR of 1642. To relate this to 'normal' life, we have to do one more sum (something called the 'Harris Benedict' formula – please don't worry about it!). If our 40-year-old female is 'sedentary' (i.e. does not take any regular exercise at all), we multiply the BMR by a factor of 1.2. So, 1642 x 1.2 = 1970 calories required for 'normal' life (let's call it 2000 calories to make the sums easier).

This is now her 'true' calorie requirement, which would allow her to maintain her current weight. *To lose weight*, she would need to eat *slightly fewer* calories or, better still, burn up more calories each day though 'activity'!

Appendix 2

More details about the foods we eat

Meat

- Much of the meat offered to us by the food industry is pretty dodgy, to be honest. For instance, a lot of the mass-produced beef in the UK involves cattle being cooped up in dark, cramped barns for large parts of the year before being fattened up on the fields for a couple of months each summer, prior to being dispatched to market.

- Although most of the beef production in this country is pretty good in terms of allowing the animals this sort of free range, they are still fed food supplements and doused with antibiotics to keep them well enough to get to market in sufficient quality to turn a profit. This is all a far cry from the sorts of meats our ancestors ate during our many thousands of years as hunter-gatherers.

- By contrast, we have some wonderful organic farmers in the UK producing ethically reared, high-quality meat at a fair price (see Appendix 3); however, there is an equally disturbing amount of evidence in the literature as to the potential health risks associated with eating red meat.

- Sadly, it seems there is a correlation between red meat consumption and certain cancers. The data is a bit 'hazy', as many of the people who appear to get ill from eating red meat also have significant other lifestyle issues too, such as smoking, alcohol abuse, heavy consumption of the burger buns and fries, together with the meat in the burgers!

- Eat natural meat (e.g. hunt your own wild game or only ever eat organic or biodynamic-produced meat) and I suspect very few of us will ever have a problem from this aspect of our diet. In fact, we will almost certainly be a lot healthier than the vast majority of the population. All in all, though, we would be better off eating vegetable proteins, organic poultry or fish in preference to most types of red meat, most of the time.

Fish

- I recommend eating certain types of fish on a regular basis. Although there have been some health concerns about the eating of fish in recent years (due mainly to fears over heavy metal content, e.g. mercury), I am more concerned about the sustainability of various fish stocks around the world.

- I eat fish and believe that if we are careful in our choices, fish provides us with a healthy and highly nutritious foodstuff. An excellent source of protein, many fish also provide high levels of very beneficial Omega 3 fatty acids.

- Don't worry too much about toxins in fish. Just stay away from the large species where these toxins might accumulate (shark, swordfish etc) and eat fish just once or twice a week. One of my favourite authors (Dr Steve Parker MD) claims to have never seen a single case of heavy metal poisoning from eating fish in his whole career!

- Nevertheless, there is no doubt that until recently, we have made a complete mess of our stewardship of the world's oceans, rivers and larger areas of fresh water. For far too long and without appropriate controls, we have treated the seas and oceans as an indiscriminate dumping ground for our waste. Because the oceans are essentially 'out of sight and out of mind', the governments of the world have in the past turned a blind eye to their care and management, leading to large-scale pollution and the dumping of garbage.

- More recently though, it appears there are grounds for optimism. Various initiatives by organizations such as the Marine Stewardship Council (www.msc.org) and effective lobbying by various NGOs etc has led to a marked improvement in policy towards managing the oceans and associated fish stocks in a much more measured and proactive manner.

- There is still a lot more to do and we can all play our part by supporting groups that advocate good stewardship of our seas and rivers etc. In the UK, I recommend you consider joining and supporting the work of the Marine Conservation Society (www.mcsuk.org) or worldwide, NGOs such as Greenpeace, Blue Ocean Institute, Oceana, The Ocean Conservancy and others, whose work is carefully focused on improving the lot of our wonderful seas and oceans.

- The world's oceans have been dramatically over-fished for decades. Stocks of some species (e.g. North Sea Cod) have almost completely collapsed due to over-fishing but the politics and economics of all this is too complex to discuss here. Nevertheless, as consumers, we can take a stand and demand that the fish we buy in the supermarkets and at the fishmongers comes from sustainable sources, which minimize the impacts on fish stocks and ease the pressure on already over-stretched fisheries around the world.

- Many of our supermarkets are making a real effort only to sell fish that comply with the MSC 'sustainable fishery' ethos. Marks and Spencer have probably taken this idea further than most but they will never be the cheapest source of fish! Nevertheless, please support these initiatives and keep the pressure on, so that efforts continue to improve the sustainability of a wide range of fisheries.

216

- Although they would rather we didn't eat fish at all (!), Greenpeace recommend the best fish to purchase in the UK are line-caught mackerel and sea bass, purse-seined herring from Cornwall and farmed mussels. In this 'online' age, I am perfectly happy to support good business that works to supply high-quality and sustainable fresh fish from around our coasts. I have no affiliation to these companies but I support both – www.fishforthought.co.uk and Wing of St Mawes (www.thecornishfishmonger.co.uk) as reliable suppliers of high-quality fish.

- Stick to salmon, mackerel and sardines etc if eating tinned fish. Make sure you look for the MSC logo to ensure, as much as we can, that the fish is from sustainable sources. Please be careful when purchasing tuna; these magnificent animals are being hunted to extinction by mass fishing, so please ensure any tuna you buy is from sustainable (and 'dolphin-friendly') sources.

- So, in summary, I think that we should eat fish in moderation, thus providing us with an excellent source of protein and 'good' fats. However, in this modern world, it is beholding on us all to ensure that we manage the oceans and their fish stocks properly, for the benefit of future generations to come. Please try to play your part by shopping for fish in a sensible, ethical manner, that's all.

Dairy products

- No other animal on this planet consumes milk other than from its mother during infancy. Humans are unique in drinking milk from other species.

- Many of us today are lactose intolerant. This is all to do with our genes, which still don't recognize the fact that we are consuming milk from another species!

- Yes, milk is full of protein and calcium, which is normally regarded as essential for good health and the avoidance of osteoporosis etc.

- However, recent research refutes this idea. For instance, the Scandinavians consume high levels of milk but have the highest rates of osteoporosis in the world! By contrast, over a billion Chinese consume no dairy but suffer from extremely low rates of osteoporosis.

- The perceived benefit of calcium intake from milk seems to be largely exaggerated. Instead, a number of vitamins are involved in calcium uptake and retention, including Vitamin D and Vitamin K, which are best obtained from exposure to sunshine (Vitamin D) and from the consumption of leafy, green vegetables (Vitamin K).

- I have no issue with a little real milk here and there,

especially if it is organic and from cows who keep their calves at foot, as Nature intended. Such enterprises now exist in the UK and will send fresh milk by courier, if you order online (e.g. www.the-calf-at-foot-dairy.co.uk). This is true, compassionate farming and a world away from the industrial production of milk, where calves are taken away from their mothers soon after birth. Real milk should not involve feeding cows grain, cereal, soya, antibiotics and other Frankenstein-style chemicals!

Eggs

- I suspect that the eggs of ground-laying birds would have provided an important source of food to our early ancestors.

- Aren't eggs full of cholesterol? Well, there is little, if any, evidence of any disease in our pre-agricultural ancestors (or modern day aboriginal communities) caused by eating eggs. Instead, much current research is firmly in the 'eggs are a cheap, natural, nutritious food that are a good source of protein and vitamins' camp, rather than the largely outdated belief that eggs contain 'bad' cholesterol.

- Most researchers now accept that the cholesterol in eggs has virtually no impact at all on blood cholesterol levels.

- I think a few eggs a week are fine; just make sure you

choose organic eggs or better still, get some chickens and have a fresh source of organic egg every morning! Please remember, though, that the risk of salmonella from eggs is still very real, so make sure you cook them properly.

Legumes

- Has evolution designed us specifically to eat legumes? Not really. Unfortunately, evolution has equipped legumes with a suite of survival chemicals that make them hard to digest for the majority of people.

- Most legumes contain a sugar called an oligosaccharide that we can't digest. This leads to a bacterial explosion in our guts as our intestinal bacterial inhabitants feed off this unexpected sugar meal, producing their own 'mini-farts' by the trillion while they tuck into their free sugary lunch. We get to pay the price down the line.

- Legumes contain various chemical 'nasties', such as our old friend lectin (which we know causes leaky gut) and phytoestrogens, which interfere with the function of certain hormones.

- I do eat some legumes and am particularly partial to Indian daal (lentils) and chickpeas prepared in numerous ways (including hummus, one of my favourite foods). However, I much prefer foods such as fruits and vegetables, fish, poultry, nuts, seeds, oils etc.

Appendix 3

Some recommended suppliers of 'real' foods!

Meats, poultry etc

- *Brown Cow Organics* (www.browncoworganics.co.uk) – one of the UK's best suppliers of organic beef. Highly recommended.
- *Heritage Prime* (www.heritageprime.co.uk) – supplies amazing biodynamic beef ('freezer' sized orders only).
- *Higher Hacknell Farm* (www.higherhacknell.co.uk) – wonderful organic poultry, beef pork and lamb. Home deliveries.
- *Laverstoke Park Farm* (www.laverstokepark.co.uk) – former racing driver Jody Scheckter's amazing biodynamic/organic farm in Hampshire. Wonderful range of products (chicken, beef etc), all home delivered.
- *Supermarkets* – most of the main supermarkets stock organic chicken etc. Do some research near your home and you will soon be able to source high-quality products.
- *Local butcher/Farmers' markets* – don't forget your local suppliers. If it proves hard to source organic poultry etc, give them a hard time until they start stocking what you want. All power to the consumer!

Fish

- *Martins Sea Fresh* (www.martins-seafresh.co.uk) – fantastic fish from Cornwall. Home deliveries.
- *Wing of St Mawes* (www.cornishfishmonger.co.uk) – another supplier of wonderful fresh seafood from Cornwall.
- *Whitby Seafish* (www.whitbyseafish.co.uk) – wonderful seafood and fish all the way from Yorkshire!
- *Swallow Fish of Seahouses* (www. swallowfish.co.uk) – great smoked salmon and kippers from Northumberland.
- *L Robson and Sons* (www.kipper.co.uk) – the finest kippers from Craster, Northumberland.
- *Various supermarkets and fish vans* – most of the better supermarkets sell good-quality fish these days. Keep your eye out for local fresh fish deliveries by the 'man in the van'. We get weekly visits from Fleetwood – great fish at reasonable prices. Find out where you buy such fish locally yourself.

Fruit and veg

Rather than list loads of suppliers here, I think it is better to locate your own local organic fruit and vegetable producer. There are suitable growers all over the country now but most only supply their local area. Join a box scheme or arrange a weekly delivery. Better still, try to grow your own!

Bibliography

Below is a list of various websites and blogs that I think are well worth a look at to learn more about the fascinating world of human nutrition. I don't necessarily agree with all or any of these authors, so please approach them with an open mind. Anyway, here is my list for your information:

Gary Taubes ('Good Calories, Bad Calories'). Gary Taubes is a highly reputable science journalist who has thrown a major spanner into the 'diet-heart' hypothesis mainstream with this groundbreaking work. In a nutshell, Taubes provides (a huge amount) of evidence as to why he believes the 'low-fat, high-carbohydrate' dogma is wrong. Instead, he suggests an altered paradigm to a diet that is low in carbohydrate, not fat. His work has influenced many doctors, researchers, authors, bloggers etc (including me) and stands as a watershed in the re-discovery of the benefits of low (processed) carb living.

Dr Jason Fung (www.intensivedietarymanagement.com). Dr Fung is a nephrologist (kidney specialist) and an expert in the treatment of obesity and Type 2 diabetes through fasting and associated dietary protocols. His writing on this subject is both very good and very popular and I highly recommend his work to those interested in learning more about the ancient art of fasting for health.

Joel Fuhrman ('Eat to Live'). Dr Fuhrman is a highly eminent medical doctor who opened my eyes to the concept of nutrient density and the benefits of his 'greens and beans' diet.

Mark Sisson (www.marksdailyapple.com). Mark Sisson is one of the leading lights in the Paleo Diet movement and his excellent blog is well worth reading on a regular basis. Mark has really thrown the spotlight on the dangers of processed carbs in particular and has done a lot to improve the health of his many online followers.

Dr Steve Parker (www.diabeticmediterraneandiet.com). One of my favourite authors, Dr Parker has published a number of books about 'low-carb Mediterranean diets' and runs an excellent blog, too. He is a highly experienced medical doctor who specializes in internal medicine and the treatment of diabetes, obesity etc.

Dr John Mericle (www.mericlediet.com). Dr Mericle is an American doctor with strong views about vegan diets and intermittent fasting. An interesting read.

Charles Dowding (www.charlesdowding.co.uk). Want to grow your own? I attended one of Charles's courses a few years ago and he remains an inspiration to those of us who want to successfully grow our own food, at home or on the local allotment. A pioneer of the 'no dig' method of vegetable growing, Charles is a mine of information and an example to us all of why we should get out in the garden and plant something! He helped me get the 'bug' for growing my own veg – there's nothing like it!

References

Introduction

1. WHO (World Health Organization) (2000). Obesity: preventing and managing the global epidemic. WHO technical report series 894.
2. Wang YC, McPherson K, Marsh T, Gortmaker SL, Brown M (2011). Health and economic burden of the projected obesity trends in the USA and the UK. *Lancet* **378**: 815–825.
3. WHO (World Health Organization) Obesity and overweight. Fact sheet N°311 Updated March 2013.
4. Health Survey for England (NS) (2015). Publication date December 14 2016.
5. Wang Y, Beydoun MA (2007). The obesity epidemic in the United States – gender, age, socioeconomic, racial/ethnic, and geographic characteristics: a systematic review and meta-regression analysis. *Epidemiol Rev* **29**: 6–28.
6. Wang Y, Beydoun MA, Liang L, Cabellero B, Kumanyika SK (2008). Will All Americans Become Overweight or Obese? Estimating the Progression and Cost of the US Obesity Epidemic. *Obesity* **16**(10): 2323–2330.
7. Whitlock G et al (2009). Body-mass index and cause-specific mortality in 900,000 adults: collaborative analyses of 57 prospective studies. *Lancet* **28**; 373 (9669).
8. Chauhan HK (2012). Diabesity: the 'Achilles Heel' of our modernized society. *Rev Assoc Med Bras* **58**(4): 399.
9. Dent M (2010). The economic burden of obesity. The National Obesity Observatory.
10. Statistics on obesity, physical activity and diet: England, 2013.

The Health and Social Care Information Centre (NHS).

11. Ogden CL, Carroll MD, Curtin LR, McDowell MA, Tabak CJ, Flegal KM (2006). Prevalence of overweight and obesity in the United States, 1999–2004. *Jama* **295**(13): 1549–55.

12. Aggarwal A, Monsivais P, Cook AJ, Drewnowski A (2011). Does diet cost mediate the relation between socioeconomic position and diet quality? *Euro J Clinical Nutrition*.

13. Brooks RC, Simpson SJ, Raubenheimer D (2010). The price of protein: combining evolutionary and economic analysis to understand excessive energy consumption. *Obes Rev* **11**(12): 887–894.

14. Prentice AM, Jebb SA (2003). Fast foods, energy density and obesity: a possible mechanistic link. *Obes Rev* **4**: 187–194.

15. Aggarwal A, Monsivais P, Cook AJ, Drewnowski A (2011). Does diet cost mediate the relation between socioeconomic position and diet quality? *Euro J Clinical Nutrition*.

Chapter 1

1. Bloch Eidner M et al (2013). Calories and portion sizes in recipes throughout 100 years: An overlooked factor in the development of overweight and obesity? *Scand J Public Health*.

2. Sikorski C et al (2012). Obese children, adults and senior citizens in the eyes of the general public: results of a representative study on stigma and causation of obesity. *PLoSOne* **7**(10) e46924.

3. Mozaffarian D et al (2011). Changes in Diet and Lifestyle and Long-Term Weight Gain in Women and Men. *N Engl J Med* **364**(25): 2392–2404.

4. Bomstein SR et al (2008). Is the worldwide epidemic of obesity a communicable feature of globalization? *Exp Clin Endocrinol Diabetes* **116**(Suppl 1):S30-2.

5. Zilberter T (2012). Food Addiction and Obesity: Do Macronutrients Matter? *Front Neuroenergetics*. 4: 7.
6. Prentice & Jebb (1995). Gluttony or sloth? *BMJ* **311**: 437.
7. Jew S et al (2009). Evolution of the human diet: linking our ancestral diet to modern functional foods as a means of chronic disease prevention. *J Med Food***12**(5): 925–34.
8. Russell-Jones D, Khan R (2007). Insulin-associated weight gain in diabetes – causes, effects and coping strategies. *Diabetes Obes Metab* **9**(6): 799–812.
9. Despres JP (1993). Abdominal obesity as important component of insulin-resistance syndrome. *Nutrition* 1993; **9**: 452–459.
10. Weiss R et al (2013). What is metabolic syndrome, and why are children getting it? *Ann NY Acad Sci* ISSN 0077-8923.
11. Frassetto LA, Schloetter M, Mietus-Synder M, Morris RC, Jr., Sebastian A (2009). Metabolic and physiologic improvements from consuming a paleolithic, hunter-gatherer type diet. *Euro J Clin Nutr* **63**(8): 947–955.
12. Newby PK, Muller D, Hallfrisch J et al (2003). Dietary patterns and changes in body mass index and waist circumference in adults. *Am J Clin Nutr* **77**: 1417–1425.

Chapter 2

1. Puhl RM et al (2013). Weight bias among professionals treating eating disorders: Attitudes about treatment and perceived patient outcomes. *Int J Eat Disord* **10**: 1002/eat.22186.
2. Vadiveloo M et al (2013). Trends in dietary fat and high-fat food intakes from 1991 to 2008 in Framingham Heart Study participants. *Br J Nutr Sep* **19**: 1–11.
3. Volger S et al (2013). Changes in eating, physical activity and related behaviors in a primary care-based weight loss intervention. *Int J Obes (Lond)* **37**(Suppl 1):S12-8.
4. Sparling PB et al (2013). Energy balance: the key to a unified

message on diet and physical activity. *J Cardiopulm Rehabil Prev* **33**(1): 12–5.

5. Buchholz AC, Schoeller DA (2004). Is a calorie a calorie? *Am J Clin Nutr* **79**(5): 899S-906S.

6. Feinman RD, Fine EJ (2004). Whatever happened to the second law of thermodynamics? *Am J Clin Nutr* **80**(5): 1445–6.

7. Schwarzfuchs D, Golan R (2012). Four-Year Follow-up after Two-Year Dietary Interventions. *N Engl J Med* **367**: 1373–1374.

8. Pereira HR et al (2013). Childhood and adolescent obesity: how many extra calories are responsible for excess of weight? *Rev Paul Paediatr* **31**(2): 252–7.

9. Slyper AH (2013). The influence of carbohydrate quality on cardiovascular disease, the metabolic syndrome, type 2 diabetes, and obesity – an overview. *J Paediatr Endocrinol Metab* **26**(7–8): 617–29.

10. Troesch B et al (2012). Dietary surveys indicate vitamin intakes below recommendations are common in representative Western countries. *Br J Nutr* **108**(4): 692–8.

11. Cizzer G, Rother KI (2012). Beyond fast food and slow motion: weighty contributors to the obesity epidemic. *J Endocrinol Invest* **35**(2): 236–42.

12. Srinivasan CS (2013). Can adherence to dietary guidelines address excess caloric intake? An empirical assessment for the UK. Econ Hum Biol S1570-677X(13)00038-5.

13. Anton S, Leeuwenburgh C (2013). Fasting or caloric restriction for Healthy Aging. *Exp Gerontol* **48**(10): 1003–5.

Chapter 3

1. Schell LM et al (2012). What's NOT to eat – Food adulteration in the context of human biology. *Am J Hum Biol* **24**(2): 139–148

2.   Diamond J (1987). The Worst Mistake In The History Of The Human Race. *Discover* 64–66.

3.   Milton K. (2002). Hunter-gatherer diets: wild foods signal relief from diseases of affluence. In: *Human Diet: Its Origins and Evolution*, Peter Ungar and Mark Teaford (eds). Westport, CT Bergin & Garvey, 111–122.

4.   Gunz P et al (2009). Early modern human diversity suggests subdivided population structure and a complex out-of-Africa scenario. *Proc Natl Acad Sci USA* **106**(15): 6094–6098.

5.   Cartmill M et al (2009). *The human lineage*. New York: John Wiley.

6.   Strait DS et al (2009). The feeding biomechanics and dietary ecology of Australopithecus africanus. *Proc Natl Acad Sci USA*. **106**(7).

7.   Tattersall I (2009). Human origins: Out of Africa. *Proc Natl Acad Sci USA*. **106**(38): 16018–16021.

8.   Wolpoff, MH, Hawks J, Frayer DW, Hunley K (2001). Modern human ancestry at the peripheries: A test of the replacement theory. *Science* **291**: 293–297.

9.   Stringer C, McKie R (1996). *African Exodus: The Origins of Modern Humanity.* New York: Henry Holt.

10.   Antón SC (2003). Natural history of Homo erectus. *Yearbook of Physical Anthropology* **46**: 126–170.

11.   Carrera-Bastos P et al (2011). The western diet and lifestyle and diseases of civilization. *Research Reports in Clinical Cardiology* **2**.

12.   McPherron SP, Alemseged Z, Marean CW, Wynn JG, Reed D, Geraads D, Bobe R, Bearat HA (2010). Evidence for stone-tool-assisted consumption of animal tissues before 3.39 million years ago at Dikika, Ethiopia. *Nature* **466**(7308): 857–860.

13.   Milton K. (2000). Back to basics: why foods of wild primates have relevance for modern human health. *Nutrition* **16**: 481-483.

14. Milton K (2000). Hunter-gatherer diets: a different perspective. *Am J Clinical Nutrition* **71**: 665–6000.

15. Chatzi L et al (2007). Protective effect of fruits, vegetables and the Mediterranean diet on asthma and allergies among children in Crete. *Thorax* **62**(8): 677–683.

16. Cordain L, Eaton SB, Sebastian A, Mann N, Lindeberg S, Watkins BA, O'Keefe JH, Brand-Miller J (2005). Origins and evolution of the western diet: Health implications for the 21st century. *Am J Clin Nutr* **81**: 341–54.

17. Diamond J et al (2003). Farmers and Their Languages: The First Expansions. *Science* **300**: 597. DOI: 10.1126/science.1078208.

18. Barrett SCH (2010). Darwin's legacy: The forms, function and sexual diversity of flowers. *Philos Trans R Soc Lond B Biol Sci* **365**(1539): 351–368.

19. De Punder K, Pruimboom L (2013). The Dietary Intake of Wheat and other Cereal Grains and Their Role in Inflammation. *Nutrients* **5**: 771–787.

20. Eaton SB (2006). The ancestral human diet: what was it and should it be a paradigm for contemporary nutrition? *Proc Nutr Soc* **65**(1): 1–6.

Chapter 4

1. Prentice & Jebb (2007). Fast foods, energy density and obesity: a possible mechanistic link. *Obesity Reviews* **4**: 187.

2. Bremer AA et al (2012). Towards a Unifying Hypothesis of Metabolic Syndrome. *Pediatrics* **129**(3): 557–570.

3. Valenzuela RER et al (2013). Insufficient amounts and inadequate distribution of dietary protein intake in apparently healthy older adults in a developing country: implications for dietary strategies to prevent sarcopenia. *Clinical Interventions in Aging* **8**.

4.   Galperin MY, Koonin UV (2012). Divergence and Convergence in Enzyme Evolution. *J Biol Chem* **287**(1): 21–28.

5.   Segasothy M, Phillips PA (1999). Vegetarian diet: panacea for modern lifestyle diseases? *QJM* **92**(9): 531–44.

6.   Martin-Peláez et al (2013). Health effects of olive oil polyphenols: recent advances and possibilities for the use of health claims. *Mol Nutr Food Res* **57**(5): 760–71.

7.   Taubes G (2008). *Good Calories, Bad Calories: Fats, carbs and the controversial science of Diet and health*. Anchor.

8.   Keys A (1970). Coronary heart disease in seven countries. Circulation 41 supplement 1: 1-1 through 1-211.

9.   Keys A (1980). *Seven countries: A multivariate analysis of death and coronary heart disease.* Harvard University Press.

10. Wainwright PE (2002). Dietary essential fatty acids and brain function: a developmental perspective on mechanisms. *Proc Nutr Soc* **61**(1): 61–9.

11. Apte SA et al (2013). A low dietary ratio of omega-6 to omega-3 Fatty acids may delay progression of prostate cancer. *Nutr Cancer* **65**(4): 556–62.

12. Simopoulos AP (2002). The importance of the ratio of omega-6/omega-3 essential fatty acids. *Biomed Pharmacother* **56**(8): 365–79.

13. Choque B et al (2013). Linoleic acid: Between doubts and certainties. *Biochimie* S0300-9084(13)00234-4.

14. Brouwer IA et al (2013).Trans fatty acids and cardiovascular health: research completed? *Euro J Clin Nutr* **67**(5): 541–7.

15. Jaworowska A et al (2013). Nutritional challenges and health implications of takeaway and fast food. *Nutr Rev* **71**(5): 310–8.

16. Catlin G (1844). Letter and notes on the Manners, Customs and Conditions of North American Indians Vol 1 and 2. Re-printed Dover Pubs NY 1971.

17. Cordain L (2006). Saturated fat consumption in ancestral human diets: implications for contemporary intakes. In:

Phytochemicals, Nutrient-Gene Interactions, Meskin MS, Bidlack WR, Randolph RK (eds). CRC Press (Taylor & Francis Group), 115-126.

18. German JB, Dillard CJ (2004). Saturated fats: what dietary intake? *Am J Clin Nutr* **80**: 550–559.

19. Forsythe CE et al (2010). Limited effect of dietary saturated fat on plasma saturated fat in the context of a low carbohydrate diet. *Lipids* **45**(10): 947–62.

20. Aranceta J, Pérez-Rodrigo C (2012). Recommended dietary reference intakes, nutritional goals and dietary guidelines for fat and fatty acids: A systematic review. *Br J Nutrition* **107**(2): S8–S22.

21. Barnard ND, Cohen J, Jenkins DJA (2006). A low-fat vegan diet improves glycemic control and cardiovascular risk factors in a randomized clinical trial in individuals with type 2 diabetes. *Diabetes Care* **29**: 1777–1783.

22. Esselstyn CB et al (2014). A way to reverse CAD? *J Fam Pract* **63**: 356–364b.

23. Barnard ND, Cohen J, Jenkins DJ et al (2009). A low-fat vegan diet and a conventional diabetes diet in the treatment of type 2 diabetes: A randomized, controlled, 74-week clinical trial. *Am J Clin Nutr* **89**: 1588S–1596S.

24. Hever J (2016). Plant-Based Diets: A Physician's Guide. *The Permanente J* **20**(3): 93–101.

25. Oyebode O et al (2014). Fruit and vegetable consumption and all-cause, cancer and CVD mortality: analysis of Health Survey for England data. *J Epidemiol Community Health Sep* **68**(9): 856–62.

26. De Souza RJ, Mente A, Maroleanu A et al (2015). Intake of saturated and trans unsaturated fatty acids and risk of all cause mortality, cardiovascular disease, and type 2 diabetes: systematic review and meta-analysis of observational studies. *BMJ* **351**: h3978.

27. Malhotra A, Redberg RF, Meier P (2017). Saturated fat does not clog the arteries: coronary heart disease is a chronic inflammatory condition, the risk of which can be effectively reduced from healthy lifestyle interventions *Br J Sports Med* 25 April.

28. Bullet Holes in Dietary Guidance (2016). The BMJ's Reputation, Stained in Scarlet. David L. Katz.

29. Dyson PA et al (2007). A low-carbohydrate diet is more effective in reducing body weight than healthy eating in both diabetic and non-diabetic subjects. *Diabet Med* **24**(12): 1430–5.

30. Feinman RD, Volek JS (2008). Carbohydrate restriction as the default treatment for type 2 diabetes and metabolic syndrome. *Scand Cardiovasc J* **42**: 256–26.

31. Aller EJG et al (2011). Starches, Sugars and Obesity. *Nutrients* **3**(3): 341–369.

32. Fuhrman J (2003). *Eat to live. The revolutionary Formula for Fast and Sustained Weight Loss.* Little Brown & Co, 1st ed.

33. Malik VS, Popkin BM, Bray GA, Després JP, Hu FB (2010). Sugar-sweetened beverages, obesity, type 2 diabetes mellitus, and cardiovascular disease risk. *Circulation* **121**(11): 1356–1364.

34. Jenkins DJ, Wolever TM, Taylor RH, Barker H, Fielden H et al (1981). Glycemic index of foods: a physiological basis for carbohydrate exchange. *Am J Clin Nutr* **34**: 362–366.

35. Barclay AW, Petocz P, McMillan-Price J et al (2008). Glycemic index, glycemic load, and chronic disease risk – a meta-analysis of observational studies. *Am J Clin Nutr* **87**: 627–637.

Chapter 5

1. Popkin BM et al (2013). NOW AND THEN: The Global Nutrition Transition: The Pandemic of Obesity in Developing Countries. *Nutr Rev* **70** (1): 3–21.

2. Williams DL, Schwarz MW (2011). Neuroanatomy of body

weight control: lessons learned from leptin. *J Clin Invest* **121**(6): 2152–2155.

3. Conte C et al (2012). Multiorgan Insulin Sensitivity in Lean and Obese Subjects. *Diabetes Care* **35**(6): 1316–1321.

4. Marlowe FW (2005). Hunter-gatherers and human evolution. *Evol Anth* **14**: 54–67.

5. Pontzer H, Raichlen DA, Wood BM, Mabulla AZP, Racette SB et al. (2012). Hunter-Gatherer Energetics and Human Obesity. *PLoS ONE* **7** (7): e40503.

6. Musselman LP et al (2011). A high-sugar diet produces obesity and insulin resistance in wild-type Drosophila. *Dis Model Mech* **4**(6): 842–849.

7. Shapiro A, Mu W, Roncal C, Cheng KY, Johnson RJ, Scarpace PJ (2008). Fructose-induced leptin resistance exacerbates weight gain in response to subsequent high-fat feeding. *Am J Physiol Regul Integr Comp Physiol* **295**: R1370–1375.

8. Taubes G (2010). *Why we get fat and what to do about it.* New York: Knopf.

9. Cizza G, Rother KI (2012). Beyond fast food and slow motion: Weighty contributors to the obesity epidemic. *J Endocrinol Invest* **35**(2): 236–242.

10. Frederich RC, Hamann A, Anderson S, Lollmann B, Lowell BB, Flier JS (1995). Leptin levels reflect body lipid content in mice: evidence for diet-induced resistance to leptin action. *Nat Med* **1**: 1311–1314.

11. Zhang Y, Proenca R, Maffei M, Barone M, Leopold L, Friedman JM (1994). Positional cloning of the mouse obese gene and its human homologue. *Nature* **372**: 425–432.

12. Aller EE et al (2011). Starches, sugars and obesity. *Nutr* **3**: 341–369.

13. Guyton AC, Hall JE (2006). Chapter 78: Insulin, Glucagon, and Diabetes Mellitus. *Textbook of Medical Physiology* (11th ed). Philadelphia: Elsevier Saunders. 963–68.

14. Kahn BB, Flier SS (2000). Obesity and insulin resistance. *J Clin Invest* **106**(4): 473–481.

15. Chakrabarti P et al (2013). Insulin Inhibits Lipolysis in Adipocytes via the Evolutionarily Conserved mTORC1-Egr1-ATGL-Mediated Pathway. *Mol Cell Biol* **33**(18): 3659–66.

16. Wilcox G (2005). Insulin and Insulin Resistance. *Clin Biochem Rev* **26**(2): 19–39.

17. El Khatib HF et al (2007). Adaptive Closed-Loop Control Provides Blood-Glucose Regulation Using Dual Subcutaneous Insulin and Glucagon Infusion in Diabetic Swine. *J Diabetes Sci Technol* **1**(2): 181–192.

18. Tsatsoulis A et al (2013). Insulin resistance: an adaptive mechanism becomes maladaptive in the current environment – an evolutionary perspective. *Metabolism* **62**(5): 622–33.

19. Ye J (2013). Mechanisms of insulin resistance in obesity. *Front Med* **7**: 14–24.

20. Kahn SE, Hull RL, Utzschneider KM (2006). Mechanisms linking obesity to insulin resistance and type 2 diabetes. *Nature* **444**: 840–846.

21. Taylor R (2013). Type 2 diabetes: etiology and reversibility. *Diabetes Care* **36**: 1047–1055.

22. Taylor R (2012). Banting Memorial lecture: Reversing the twin cycles of type 2 diabetes. *Diabet Med* **30**: 267–275.

23. Hruby A, Hu FB (2015). The Epidemiology of Obesity: A Big Picture. *Pharmacoeconomics* **33**: 673–689.

24. Al-Mrabeh A, Hollingsworth KG, Steven S, Tiniakos D, Taylor R (2017). Quantification of intrapancreatic fat in type 2 diabetes by MRI. *PLoS ONE* **12**(4): e0174660.

25. Wilding JP (2014). The importance of weight management in type 2 diabetes mellitus. *Int J Clin Pract* **68**(6): 682–691.

26. Hansen M, Chandra A, Mitic LL, Onken B, Driscoll M, Kenyon C (2008). A role for autophagy in the extension of

lifespan by dietary restriction in Caenorhabditis elegans. *PLoS Genetics* **4**(2): e24.

27. Hsu AL, Murphy CT, Kenyon C (2003). Regulation of aging and age-related disease by DAF-16 and Heat-Shock Factor. *Science* **300**(5622): 1142–1145.

28. Kui Lin, Hsin H, Libina N, Kenyon C (2001). Regulation of the Caenorhabditis elegans longevity protein DAF-16 by insulin/IGF-1 and germline signaling. *Nature Genetics* **28**(2): 139–145.

Chapter 6

1. http://www.livestrong.com/article/40956-six-small-meals-day-diet/

2. Cameron JD, Cyr MJ, Doucet E (2010). Increased meal frequency does not promote greater weight loss in subjects who were prescribed an 8-week equi-energetic energy-restricted diet. *Br J Nutr* **103**(8): 1098–101.

3. DeBerardinis RJ, Craig BT (2012). Cellular metabolism and disease: what do metabolic outliers teach us? *Cell* **148**(6): 1132–1144.

4. Solomon TPJ et al (2008). The effect of feeding frequency on insulin and ghrelin responses in human subjects. *Br J Nutrition* **100**: 810–819.

5. Oh KJ et al (2013). Transcriptional regulators of hepatic gluconeogenesis. *Arch Pharm Res* **36**(2): 189–200.

6. Nishino N et al (2007). Insulin Efficiently Stores Triglycerides in Adipocytes by Inhibiting Lipolysis and Repressing PGC-1 Induction. *Kobe J Med Sci* **53**(3): 99–106

7. Bonadonna RC, Groop LC, Zych K, Shank M, DeFronzo RA (1990). Dose-dependent effect of insulin on plasma free fatty acid turnover and oxidation in humans. *Am J Physiol* **259**(Endocrinol. Metab. 22): E736–E750.

8. Campbell PJ, Carlson MG, Hill JO, Nurjhan N (1992). Regulation of free fatty acid metabolism by insulin in humans: role of lipolysis and reesterification. *Am J Physiol* **263**(Endocrinol. Metab. 26): E1063–E1069.

9. Berg JM, Tymoczko JL, Stryer L (2002). *Biochemistry*, 5th ed. New York: W H Freeman.

10. Chambliss HO (2005). Exercise duration and intensity in a weight-loss program. *Clin J Sport Med***15**(2): 113–5.

11. Jason Fung MD, Moore J (2016). *The complete guide to fasting.* (1st ed) Las Vegas: Victory Belt Publishing.

12. Jason Fung MD (2016). *The Obesity Code* (1st ed). Greystone.

13. Nematy M et al (2012). Effects of Ramadan fasting on cardiovascular risk factors: a prospective observational study. *Nutr J* **11**: 69.

14. Shariatpanahi ZV, Shariatpanahi MV, Shahbazi S, Hossaini A, Abadi A (2008). Effect of Ramadan fasting on some indices of insulin resistance and components of the metabolic syndrome in healthy male adults. *Br J Nutr* **100**(1): 147–151.

15. Bouguerra R, Jabrane J, Maatki C, Ben SL, Hamzaoui J, El KA et al (2006). Ramadan fasting in type 2 diabetes mellitus. *Ann Endocrinol* **67**(1): 54–59.

16. Halberg N, Henriksen M, Soderhamn N, Stallknecht B, Ploug T, Schjerling P et al. (2005). Effect of intermittent fasting and refeeding on insulin action in healthy men. *J Appl Physiol* **99**(6): 2128–2136.

17. Keogh JB, Pedersen E, Petersen KS, Clifton PM (2014). Effects of intermittent compared to continuous energy restriction on short-term weight loss and long-term weight loss maintenance. *Clin Obes* **4**: 150–156.

Chapter 7

1. Ravnskov U (1998). The questionable role of saturated and

polyunsaturated fatty acids in cardiovascular disease. *J Clin Epidemiol* **51**: 443–460.

2. Pavitt N (1997). *Turkana*. London: Harvill Press.

3. Lindeberg S, Nilsson-Ehle P, Terént A, Vessby B, Scherstén B (1994). Cardiovascular risk factors in a Melanesian population apparently free from stroke and ischaemic heart disease – the Kitava study. *J Intern Med* **236**: 331–340.

4. Popkin BM, Adair LS, Ng SW (2012). Global nutrition transition and the pandemic of obesity in developing countries. *Nutr Rev* **70**: 3-21.

5. Zheng W et al (2011). Association between body-mass index and risk of death in more than 1 million Asians. *N Engl J Med* **364**(8): 719–729.

6. Mehio Sibai A, Nasreddine L, Mokdad AH, Adra N, Tabet M, Hwalla N (2010). Nutrition transition and cardiovascular disease risk factors in Middle East and North Africa countries: reviewing the evidence. *Ann Nutr Metab* **57**(3–4).

7. Volek JS (2012). Carbohydrate restriction uniquely benefits metabolic syndrome and saturated fat metabolism. *BMC Proc* **6**(Suppl 3).

8. Spreadbury I (2012). Comparison with ancestral diets suggests dense acellular carbohydrates promote an inflammatory microbiota, and may be the primary dietary cause of leptin resistance and obesity. *Diabetes Metab Syndr Obes* **5**: 175–89.

9. Lindeberg S, Soderberg S, Ahren B, Olsson T (2001). Large differences in serum leptin levels between nonwesternized and westernized populations: the Kitava study. *J Intern Med* **249**(6): 553–558.

10. Frassetto LA, Schloetter M, Mietus-Synder M, Morris RC Jr, Sebastian A (2009). Metabolic and physiologic improvements from consuming a paleolithic, hunter-gatherer type diet. *Eur J Clin Nutr* 63(8): 947–955.

11. Lassenius MI, Pietilainen KH, Kaartinen K et al (2011). Bacterial endotoxin activity in human serum is associated with dyslipidemia, insulin resistance, obesity, and chronic inflammation. *Diabetes Care* **34**(8): 1809–1815.

12. Berry E, Arnoni Y, Aviram M (2011). The middle-eastern & biblical origins of the Mediterranean diet. *Public Health Nutr* **14**(12A).

13. Ancel Keys (ed) (1980). *Seven Countries: A multivariate analysis of death and coronary heart disease,*. Cambridge, Mass.: Harvard University Press.

14. Anderson JJB, Nieman DC (2016). Diet Quality – The Greeks Had It Right! *Nutrients* **8**(10): 636.

15. Trichopoulou A et al (2014). Definitions and potential health benefits of the Mediterranean diet: Views from experts around the world. *BMC Med* **12**: 112–128.

16. Estruch R et al (2013). PREDIMED Study Investigators Primary prevention of cardiovascular disease with a Mediterranean diet. *N Engl J Med* **368**: 1279–1290.

17. Di Daniele N et al (2017). Impact of Mediterranean diet on metabolic syndrome, cancer and longevity. *Oncotarget* **8**(5): 8947–8979.

18. Romaguera D et al (2010). Mediterranean dietary patterns and prospective weight change in participants of the EPIC-PANACEA project. *Am J Clin Nutr* **92**: 912–921.

19. Martínez-González MA et al (2012). The PREDIMED Trial. Peiró C, ed. *PLoS ONE.* **7**(8): e43134.

20. Mozaffarian D (2016). Dietary and Policy Priorities for Cardiovascular Disease, Diabetes, and Obesity – A Comprehensive Review. *Circulation* **133**(2): 187–225.

21. Cicerale S, Lucas L, Keast R (2010). Biological Activities of Phenolic Compounds Present in Virgin Olive Oil. *Int J Molecular Sci* **11**(2): 458–479.

22. Balakireva AV, Zamyatnin AA (2016). Properties of Gluten

Intolerance: Gluten Structure, Evolution, Pathogenicity and Detoxification Capabilities. *Nutrients*. **8**(10): 644.

23. Springmann M et al (2016). Analysis and valuation of the health and climate change cobenefits of dietary change. *Proc Nat Acad Sci USA* **113**(15): 4146–4151.

24. Perignon M et al (2017). Improving diet sustainability through evolution of food choices: review of epidemiological studies on the environmental impact of diets. *Nutrition Reviews* **75**(1): 2–17.

25. Joyce A, Dixon S, Comfort J, Hallett J (2012). Reducing the Environmental Impact of Dietary Choice: Perspectives from a Behavioural and Social Change Approach. *J Environmental and Public Health* **20**12: 978672.

26. Macdiarmid JI, Douglas F, Campbell J (2016). Eating like there's no tomorrow: Public awareness of the environmental impact of food and reluctance to eat less meat as part of a sustainable diet. *Appetite* **96**: 487–493.

27. Le LT, Sabaté J (2014). Beyond meatless, the health effects of vegan diets: Findings from the adventist cohorts. *Nutrients* **6**: 2131–2147.

28. Huang R-Y, Huang C-C, Hu FB, Chavarro JE (2016). Vegetarian Diets and Weight Reduction: a Meta-Analysis of Randomized Controlled Trials. *J General Internal Medicine* **31**(1): 109-116.

29. Lee Y-M, Kim S-A, Lee I-K et al (2016). Effect of a Brown Rice Based Vegan Diet and Conventional Diabetic Diet on Glycemic Control of Patients with Type 2 Diabetes: A 12-Week Randomized Clinical Trial. Meyre D, ed. *PLoS ONE*. **11**(6).

30. Barnard ND et al (2009). A low-fat vegan diet elicits greater macronutrient changes, but is comparable in adherence and acceptability, compared with a more conventional diabetes diet among individuals with type 2 diabetes. *J Am Diet Assoc* **109**: 263–272.

31. Glick-Bauer M, Yeh M-C (2014). The Health Advantage of a Vegan Diet: Exploring the Gut Microbiota Connection. *Nutrients* **6**(11): 4822–4838.

32. Craig WJ (2009). Health effects of vegan diets. *Am J Clin Nutr* **89**: 1627S–1633S.

Some extra 'fruit and veg' references (see page 59)

1. Agudo A, Slimani N, Ocké MC et al (2002). Consumption of vegetables, fruit and other plant foods in the European prospective investigation into cancer and nutrition (EPIC) cohorts from 10 European countries. *Public Health Nutr* **5**: 1179–1196.

2. Alinia S, Hels O, Tetens I (2009). The potential association between fruit intake and body weight – a review. *Obes Rev* **10**: 639–647.

3. Appleby PN, Thorogood M, Mann JI, Key TJ (1999). The Oxford Vegetarian Study: an overview. *Am J Clin Nutr* **70**(3 Suppl): 525S–531S

4. Bazzano LA (2005). *Dietary intake of fruits and vegetables and risk of diabetes mellitus and cardiovascular disease.* World Health Organization, Geneva.

5. Bendinelli B, Masala G, Saieva C et al (2011). Fruit, vegetables, and olive oil and risk of coronary heart disease in Italian women: the EPICOR Study. *Am J Clin Nutr* **93**: 275–283.

6. Block G, Patterson B, Subar A (1992). Fruit, vegetables, and cancer prevention: a review of the epidemiological evidence. *Nutr Cancer* **18**: 29.

7. Boffetta P, Couto E, Wichmann J et al (2010). Fruit and vegetable intake and overall cancer risk in the European Prospective Investigation into Cancer and Nutrition (EPIC) *J Natl Cancer Inst* **102**: 529–537.

8. Buijsse B, Feskens EJ, Schulze MB et al (2009). Fruit and

vegetable intakes and subsequent changes in body weight in European populations: results from the project on diet, obesity, and genes (DiOGenes). *Am J Clin Nutr* **90**: 202–209

9.   Carter P, Gray LJ, Troughton J et al (2010). Fruit and vegetable intake and incidence of type 2 diabetes mellitus: systematic review and meta-analysis. *BMJ* **341**: c4229.

10.   Crowe FL, Roddam AW, Key TJ et al (2011). European prospective investigation into cancer and nutrition (EPIC)-heart study collaborators. Fruit and vegetable intake and mortality from ischaemic heart disease: results from the European Prospective Investigation into Cancer and Nutrition (EPIC)-Heart Study. *Eur Heart . ***32**: 1235–1243.

11.   Dauchet L, Amouyel P, Dallongeville J (2005). Fruit and vegetable consumption and risk of stroke: a metaanalysis of cohort studies. *Neurology* **65**: 1193–1197.

12.   Dauchet L, Amouyel P, Hercberg S, Dallongeville J (2006). Fruit and vegetable consumption and risk of coronary heart disease: a meta-analysis of cohort studies. *J Nutr* **136**: 2588–2593.

13.   Davey GK, Spencer EA, Appleby PN, Allen NE, Knox KH, Key TJ (2003). EPIC-Oxford: lifestyle characteristics and nutrient intakes in a cohort of 33 883 meat-eaters and 31 546 non meat-eaters in the UK. *Public Health Nutr* **6**: 259–269

14.   Erlund I, Koli R, Alfthan G et al (2007). Favourable effects of berry consumption on platelet function, blood pressure, and HDL cholesterol. *Am J Clin Nutr* **87**: 323–331

15.   Field AE, Gillman MW, Rockett HR, Colditz GA (2003). Association between fruit and vegetable intake and change in body mass index among a large sample of children and adolescents in the United States. *Int J Obes* **27**: 821–826.

16.   George SM, Park Y, Leitzmann MF et al (2009). Fruit and vegetable intake and risk of cancer: a prospective cohort study. *Am J Clin Nutr* **89**: 347–353.

17.   Hall JN, Moore S, Harper SB, Lynch JW (2009). Global

variability in fruit and vegetable consumption. *Am J Prev Med* **36**: 402–409.

18. Hamer M, Chida Y (2007). Intake of fruit, vegetables, and antioxidants and risk of type 2 diabetes: systematic review and meta-analysis. *J Hypertens* **25**: 2361–2369.

19. Hamidi M, Boucher BA, Cheung AM et al (2011). Fruit and vegetable intake and bone health in women aged 45 years and over: a systematic review. *Osteoporos Int.* **22**: 1681–1693.

20. Harding AH, Wareham NJ, Bingham SA et al (2008). Plasma vitamin C level, fruit and vegetable consumption, and the risk of new-onset type 2 diabetes mellitus: the European prospective investigation of cancer – Norfolk prospective study. *Arch Intern Med* **168**: 1493–1499.

21. He FJ, Nowson CA, MacGregor GA (2006). Fruit and vegetable consumption and stroke: meta-analysis of cohort studies. *Lancet* **367**: 320–326.

22. He FJ, Nowson CA, Lucas M, Macgregor GA (2007). Increased consumption of fruit and vegetables is related to a reduced risk of coronary heart disease: meta-analysis of cohort studies. *J Hum Hypertens* **21**: 717–728.

23. Hoffmann K, Boeing H, Volatier JL, Becker W (2003). Evaluating the potential health gain of the World Health Organization's recommendation concerning vegetable and fruit consumption. *Public Health Nutr* **6**: 765–772.

24. Hung HC, Joshipura KJ, Jiang R et al (2004). Fruit and vegetable intake and risk of major chronic disease. *J Nat Cancer Inst.* **96**: 1577–1584.

25. John JH, Ziebland S, Yudkin P et al (2002). Effects of fruit and vegetable consumption on plasma antioxidant concentrations and blood pressure: a randomised controlled trial. *Lancet* **359**: 1969–1974.

26. Key TJ (2011). Fruit and vegetables and cancer risk. *Br J Cancer* **104**: 6–11.

27. Nuñez-Cordoba JM, Alonso A, Beunza JJ et al (2002). Role of vegetables and fruits in Mediterranean diets to prevent hypertension. *Eur J Clin Nutr* **63**: 605–612.

28. Riboli E, Norat T (2003). Epidemiologic evidence of the protective effect of fruit and vegetables on cancer risk. *Am J Clin Nutr* **78**: 559S–569S.

29. Rolls BJ, Ello-Martin JA, Tohill BC (2004). What can intervention studies tell us about the relationship between fruit and vegetable consumption and weight management? *Nutr Rev* **62**: 1–17.

30. Zino S, Skeaff M, Williams S, Mann J (1997). Randomised controlled trial of effect of fruit and vegetable consumption on plasma concentrations of lipids and antioxidants. *BMJ* **314**: 1787–1791.